PRECLINICAL DENTAL SCIENCES

PRECLINICAL DENTAL SCIENCES
PRECLINICAL DENTAL SCIENCES

WORKBOOK FOR DENTAL STUDENTS

PRECLINICAL DENTAL SCIENCES

WORKBOOK FOR DENTAL STUDENTS

KEFI IQBAL
Ph.D. (PK), M.Sc (London), B.D.S (KU)
Professor and Head, Department of Science of Dental Materials
Baqai Dental College
Baqai Medical University
Karachi, Pakistan

©
Paramount Books (Pvt.) Ltd.
Karachi | Lahore | Islamabad | Hyderabad | Faisalabad | Peshawar | Abbottabad

Preclinical Dental Sciences

by

Kefi Iqbal

Medical knowledge is constantly changing. As new information becomes available, changes in treatment, procedures, equipment and the use of drugs become necessary. The editors, contributors and the publishers have, as far as it is possible, taken care to ensure that the information given in this text is accurate and up-to-date. However, readers are strongly advised to confirm that the information, especially with regard to drug usage, complies with the latest legislation and standards of practice.

First Edition 2014

Reprint 2015

Paramount Books (Pvt.) Ltd.

152/O, Block-2, P.E.C.H.S., Karachi-75400. Tel: 34310030
Fax: 34553772, E-mail: info@paramountbooks.com.pk
Website: www.paramountbooks.com.pk

ISBN: 978-969-494-975-8
Printed in Pakistan

Dedicated

To my dear students for their love and care

PROFORMA FOR DENTAL STUDENTS

paste photo here

Year 20_____

CLASS ROLL NO: ________________ EXAM SEAT NO: ____________________

NAME: ____

ADDRESS: ____

____

PHONE(RES): ____________________________________ CELL: ____

EMAIL ADDRESS: ____

FATHERS/GUARDIANS NAME: ____

PHONE(RES): ______________________ PHONE(OFF): ____________________ CELL: ______________________

ADDRESS OF PARENTS/GUARDIANS: ____

____

SIGNATURE OF STUDENT: ____

PRACTICAL EVALUATION RECORD

PRACTICAL WORK

WORK BOOK	***TOTAL MARKS***	***MARKS OBTAINED***

PRACTICAL ATTENDANCE

TOTAL NUMBER OF PRACTICALS	***ATTENDANCE***	***%AGE***

HEAD OF THE DEPARTMENT REMARKS:

____

____

____

REQUIREMENTS FOR PRACTICAL COURSE

INSTRUMENTS

A: FOR WIRE BENDING WORK

(1)- Pliers

1. Round Plier
2. Flat Plier
3. Wire Cutter
4. Adam's Plier

(2)- Wire (Stainless Steel/Gauge: 0.7 mm)

B: FOR WAX UP AND TEETH ARRANGEMENT

1. Wax Knife
2. Wax Carver
3. Spirit Lamp
4. Glass Slab (6″ X 6″)
5. Instrument Tray
6. Aluminium Foil Sheet
7. Plastic Sheet

C: FOR PLASTER SLAB/BLOCK MAKING

1. Rubber Bowl
2. Plaster Spatula
3. Straight End Spatula
4. Plaster Knife
5. Glass Slab

D: STATIONERY REQUIRED

1. Black Pointer
2. Pencil
3. Scale
4. Marker
5. China Graph Pencil

LAB PROTOCOLS

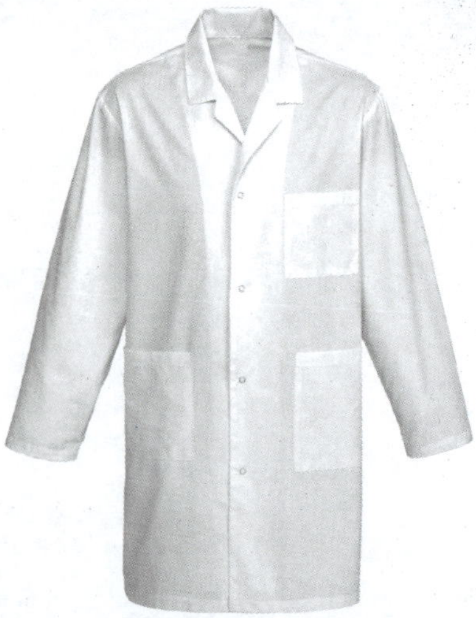

Lab Coat

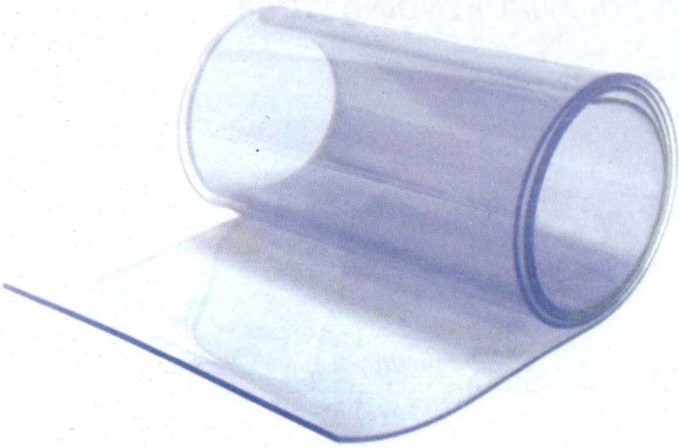

Plastic Sheet

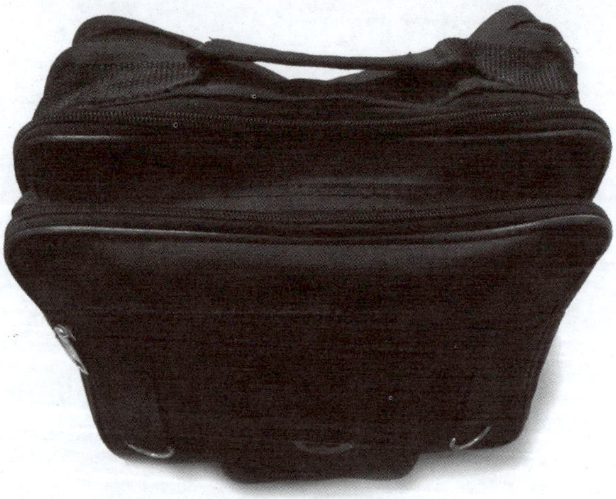

Practical Instruments Kit

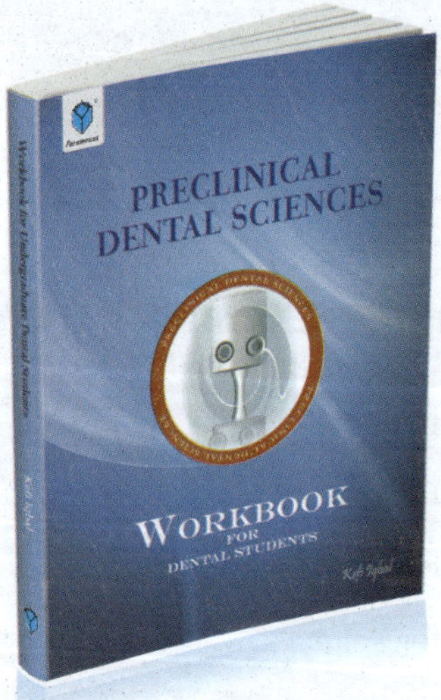

Practical Workbook

Note:

No Entrance Without Lab Protocols

CONTENTS

INSTRUCTOR REMARKS

Date	Practical #	Remarks	Initials
	1		
	2		
	3		
	4		
	5		
	6		
	7		
	8		
	9		
	10		
	11		
	12		
	13		
	14		

Note:

A^+ = Excellent

A = V. Good

B = Good

B^+ = Fair

C = Average

D = Below average

FOREWORD

Preclinical Dental Sciences is a very dynamic and important discipline not only for the students but also for practitioners of Dental Sciences.

This practical workbook is designed to introduce students to various dental materials used in clinical and laboratory techniques. This logbook denotes the input of compilation of Student's activities in the practical session. This book will be a guide to the students towards completion of their assignments, which include wax up, teeth setup, clasp making for acrylic partial dentures, wire bending, making plaster slabs and attending demonstrations on the steps on fabrication of partial dentures and complete dentures.

The practical part of this work book provides practical hands on, problem based learning and the correlation of the materials taught in theoretical part of this subject.

Each student has to complete this logbook, get it signed by the Supervisor and Head of the Department and submit it before final examination.

On behalf of Department of Science of Dental Materials, I wish you an enjoyable and productive time during your studies of this practical course.

Being a initial learner, your effort, commitment and continuous work will help to achieve your goal by applying your skills, regularity and self evaluation of your performance.

The Department, acknowledges the team work and cooperation of all the faculty members whose valuable efforts made the preparation of the logbook possible.

Prof. Dr. Kefi Iqbal

CONTRIBUTORS

Dr Adel Zia Siddiqui
B.D.S (KU), M.Sc (London)
Assistant Professor
Department of Science of Dental Materials
Baqai Dental College
Baqai Medical University
Karachi

Dr Maria Asmat
B.D.S (BMU), R.D.S
Senior Lecturer
Department of Science of Dental Materials
Baqai Dental College
Baqai Medical University
Karachi

Dr Afreen Mushtaq
B.D.S (HU), R.D.S
Demonstrator
Department of Science of Dental Materials
Baqai Dental College
Baqai Medical University
Karachi

Dr Sana Jawed
B.D.S (BMU), R.D.S
Demonstrator
Department of Science of Dental Materials
Baqai Dental College
Baqai Medical University
Karachi

Dr Muhammad Kaleem
B.D.S (Pb), M.Sc (London), Ph.D. (Manchester)
Assistant Professor and Head of the Department
Department of Science of Dental Materials
Army Medical College
National University of Science and Technology
Islamabad

Dr Naresh Kumar
B.D.S (Sindh), Ph.D. (Birmingham)
Assistant Professor and Head of the Department
Department of Science of Dental Materials
Liaquat University of Medical and Health Sciences
Hyderabad

Dr Amber Fareed
B.D.S (Pb), M.Sc (London), Ph.D. (Birmingham)
Assistant Professor and Head of the Department
Department of Science of Dental Materials
Nur Centre for Research & Policy
Room# 19, 4th Floor, College Building
Fatima Memorial Hospital Shadman
Lahore

Section A

WIRE BENDING

1
PRACTICAL

ALPHABET 'A'

Grading

Date : ____________________

Grade : ____________________

Sign : ____________________

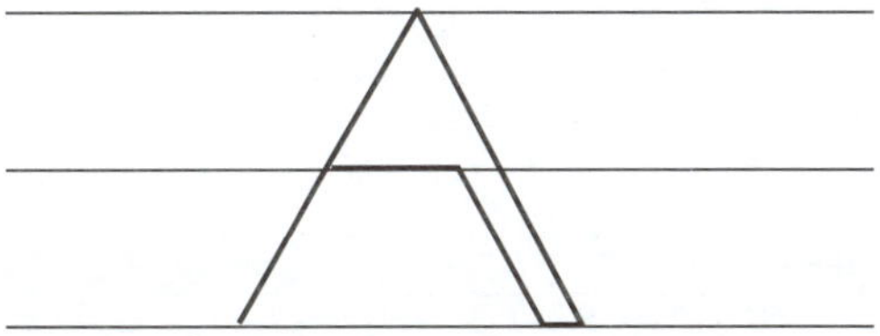

Date : ____________________

Grade : ____________________

Sign : ____________________

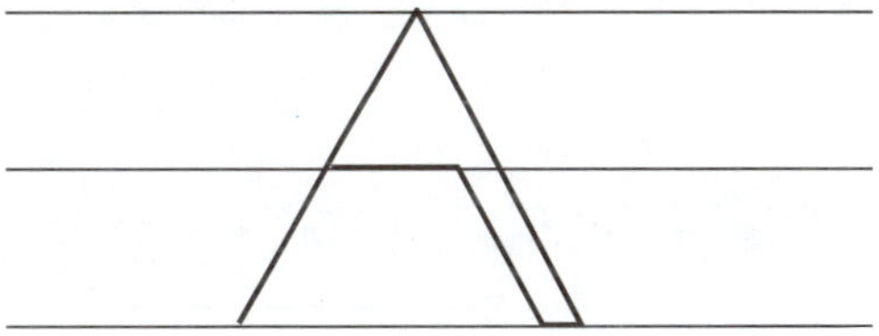

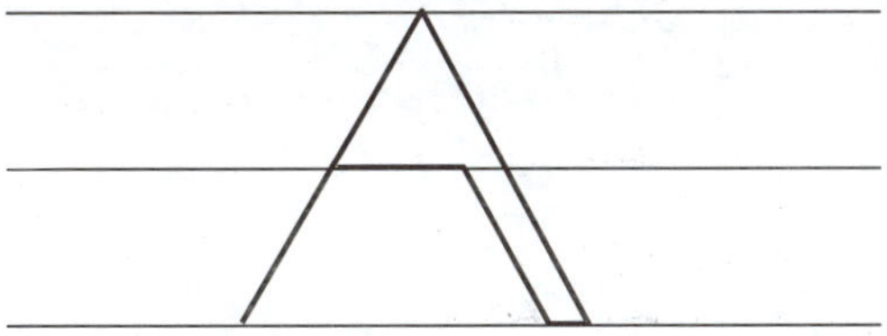

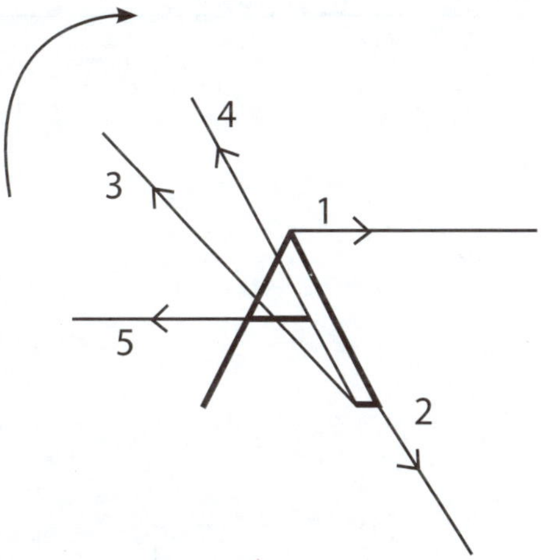

ALPHABET 'B'

Grading

Date : ____________________

Grade : ____________________

Sign : ____________________

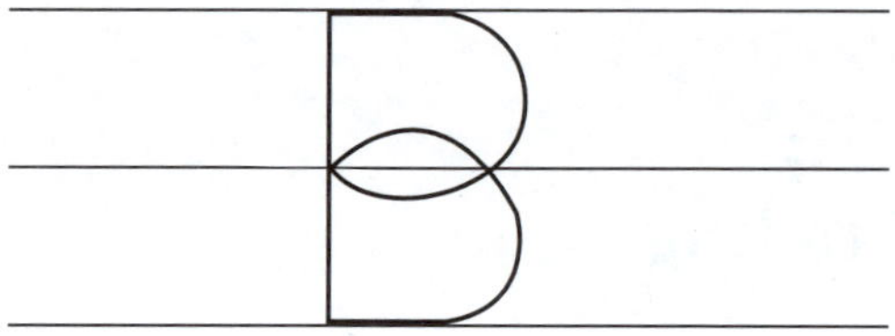

Date : ____________________

Grade : ____________________

Sign : ____________________

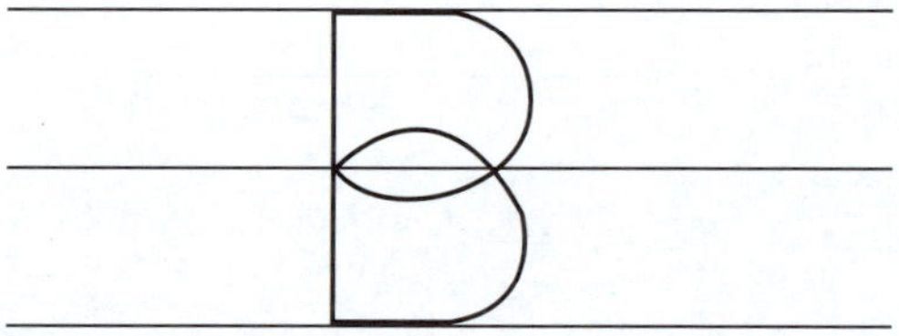

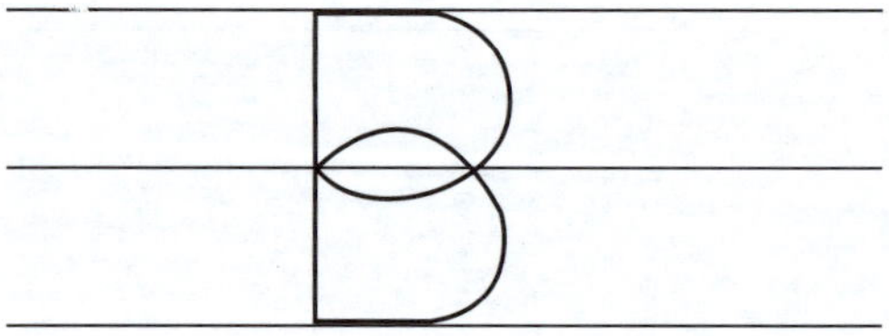

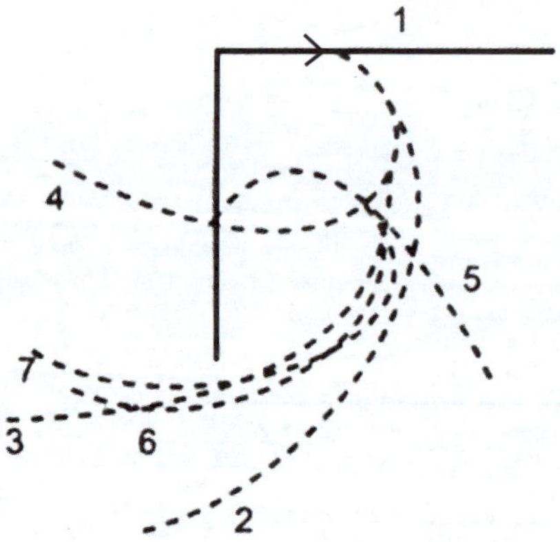

ALPHABET 'G'

Grading

Date : ____________________

Grade : ____________________

Sign : ____________________

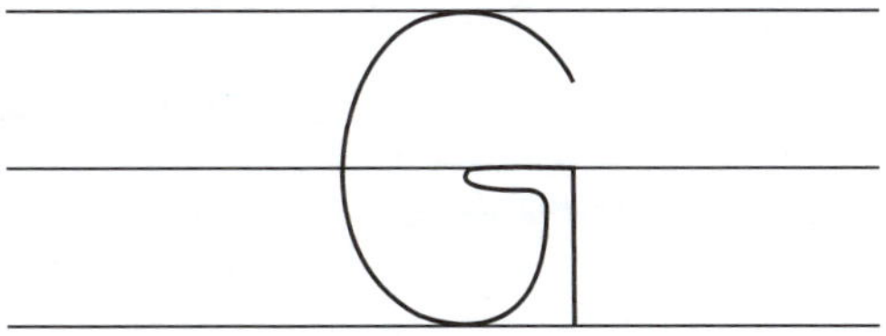

Date : ____________________

Grade : ____________________

Sign : ____________________

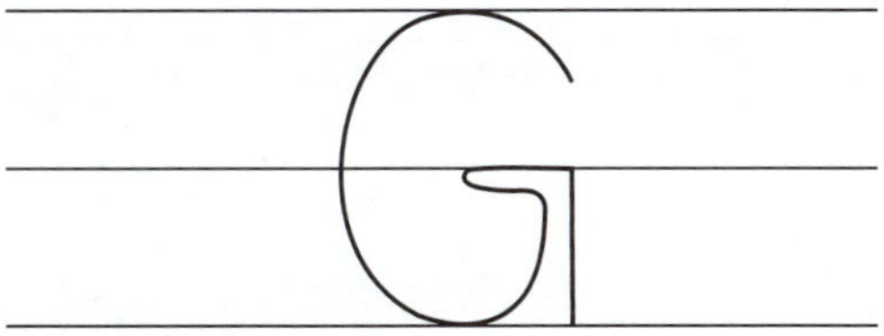

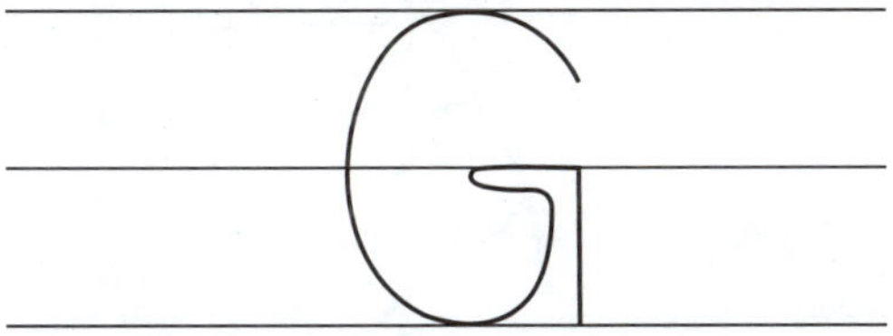

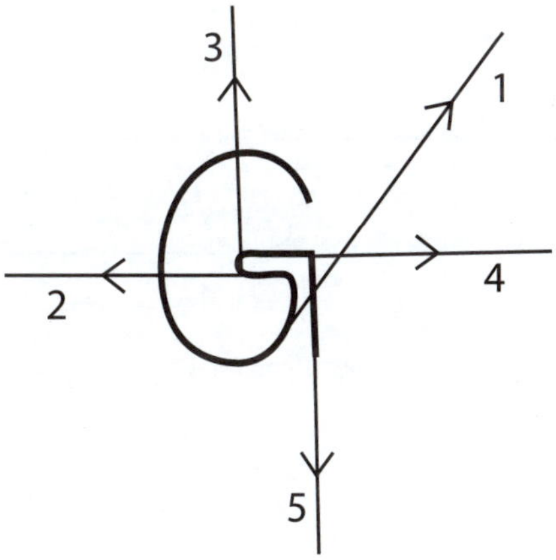

ALPHABET 'S'

Grading

Date : ____________________

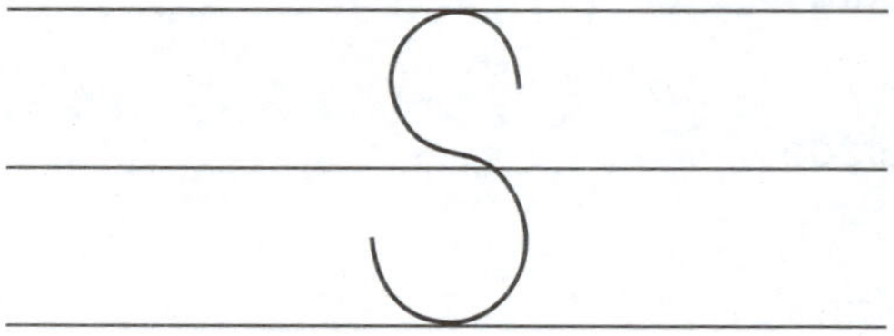

Grade : ____________________

Sign : ____________________

Date : ____________________

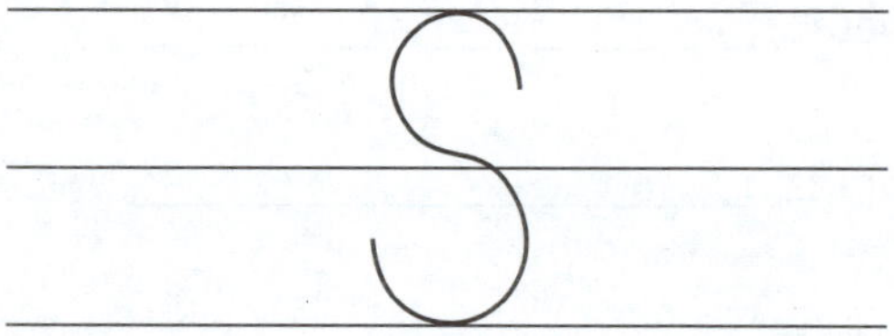

Grade : ____________________

Sign : ____________________

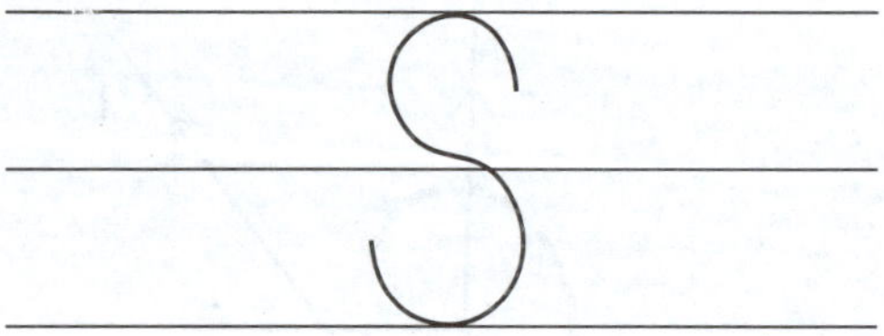

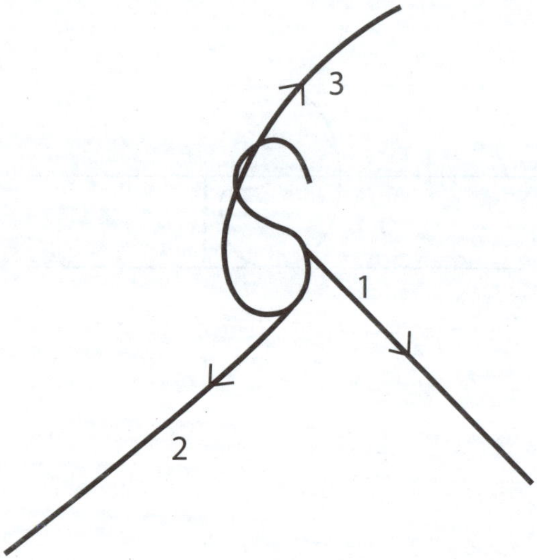

FABRICATION OF ADAM'S CLASP

2
PRACTICAL

STEPS OF ADAM'S CLASP

1

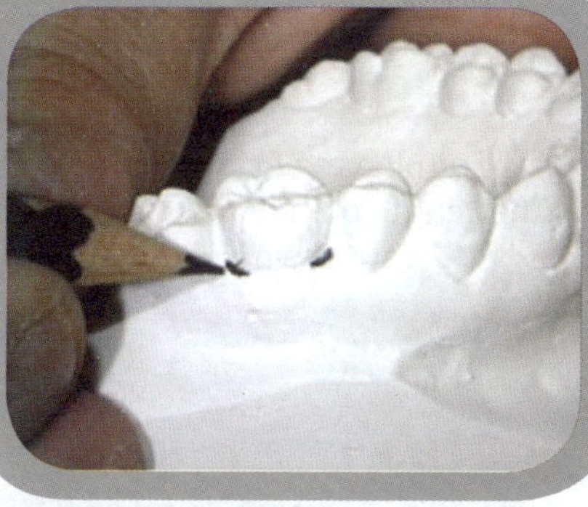

Mark Position of Mesial and
Distal Undercuts

2

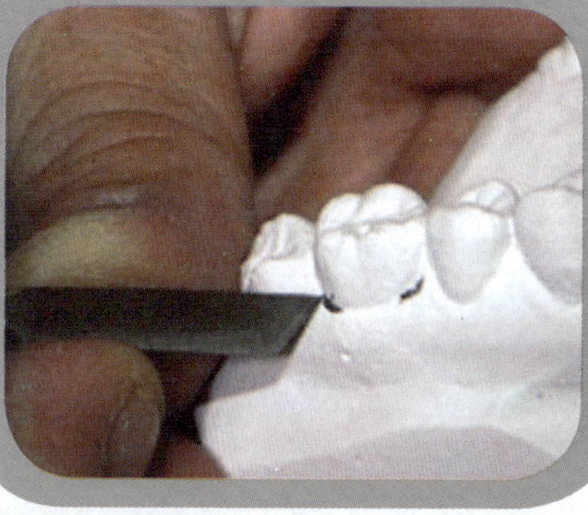

Prepare Undercuts.
These Should be Prepared to Approx. 1mm in
Depth. Avoid Trimming the Buccal Surface of Tooth

3

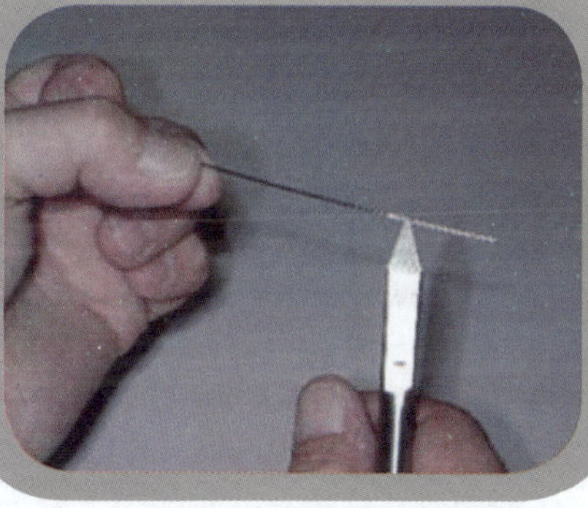

Straighten a Piece of 0.7mm
Stainless Steel Wire

4

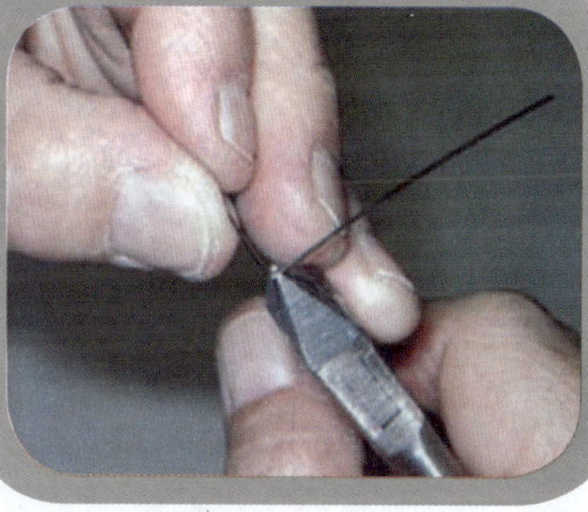

Make a 90° Bend

5

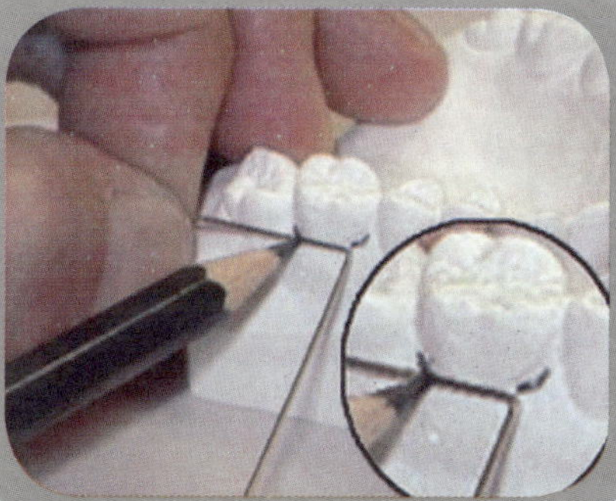

Mark the Length of the Bridge on to the Wire.
This Should be the Distance Between the Two
Marks on the Model Where the Arrowheads
Will Engage the Undercuts

6

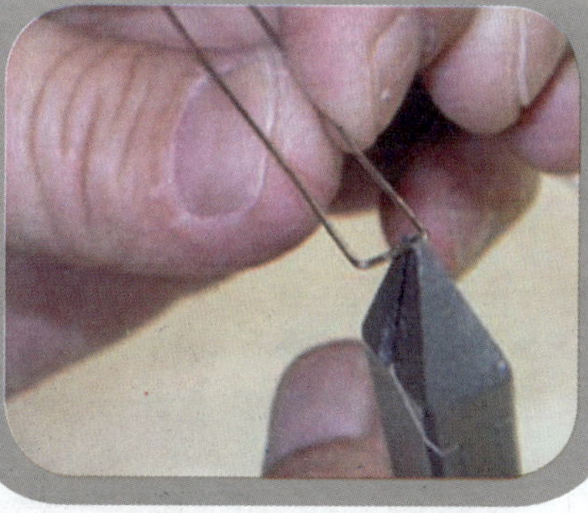

Make Another 90° Bend

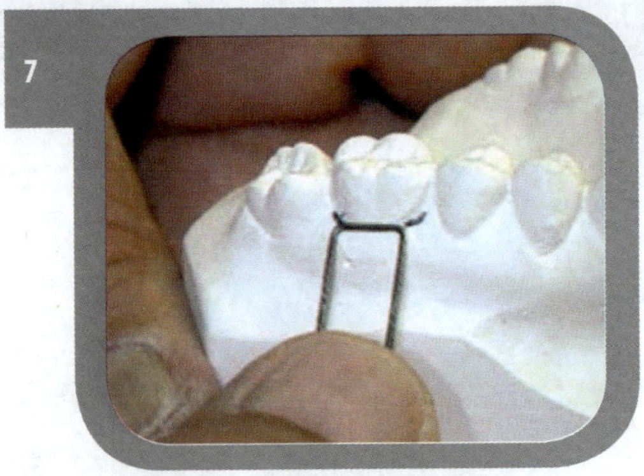

Check Length of Bridge
Against Model

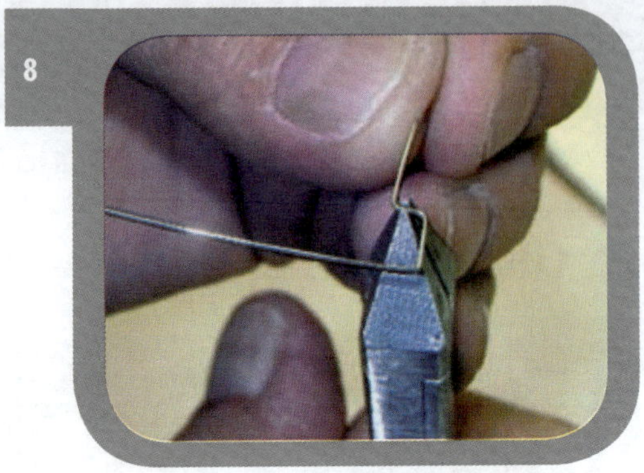

Forming the Arrowhead's First Bend.
The Length of the Arrowhead is Determined
by Crown Height of Tooth

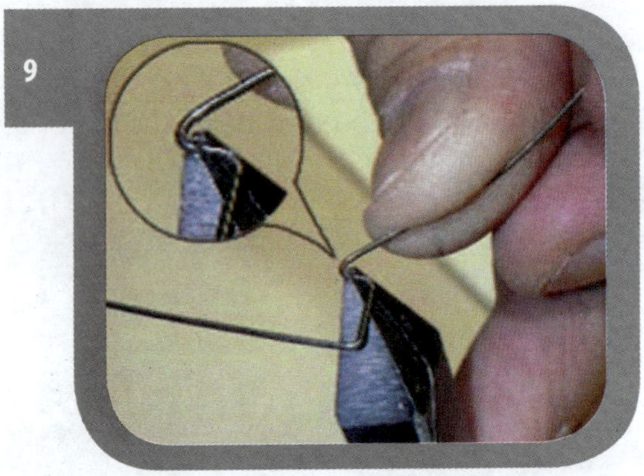

Forming the Arrowhead's First Bend.
The Length of the Arrowhead is Determined
by Crown Height of Tooth

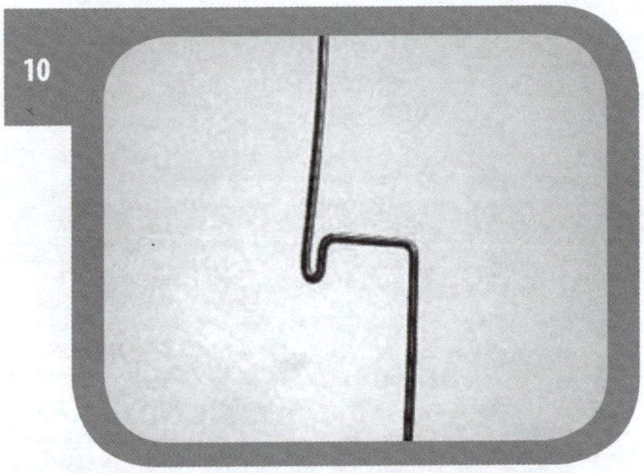

First Arrowhead Formed.
Both Sides of Arrowhead Should be Parallel.
First Bend into Arrowhead Should be 90° to Bridge

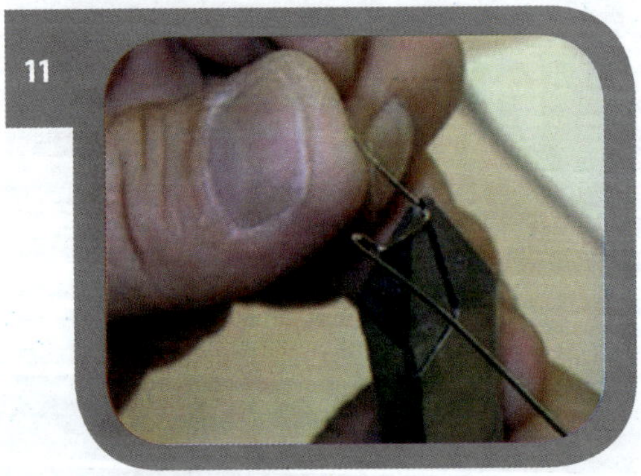

Forming Second Arrowhead

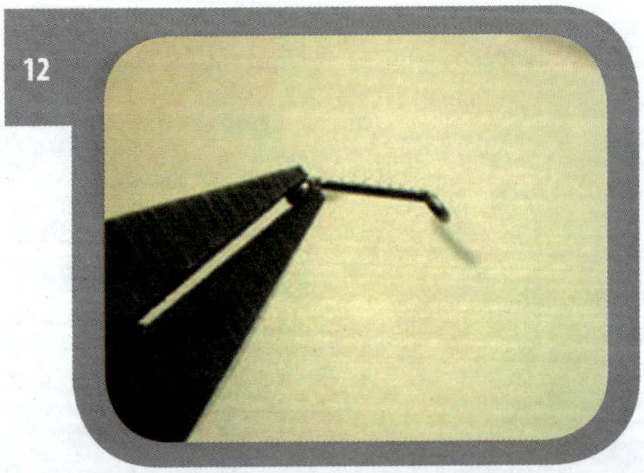

Arrowheads are Angled to
Follow Tooth Contours

13

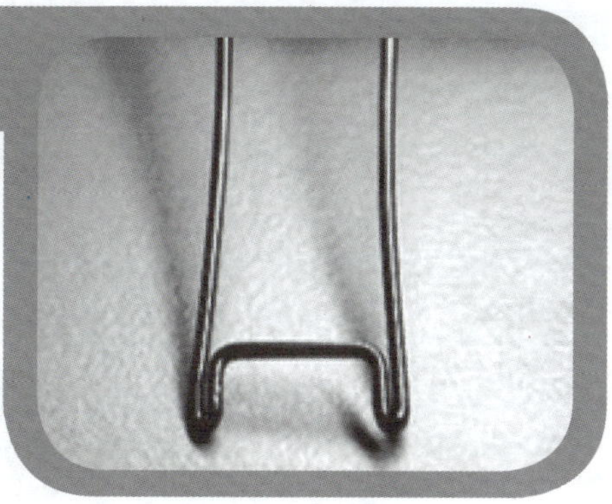

Check Angles and Arrowheads are Parallel

14

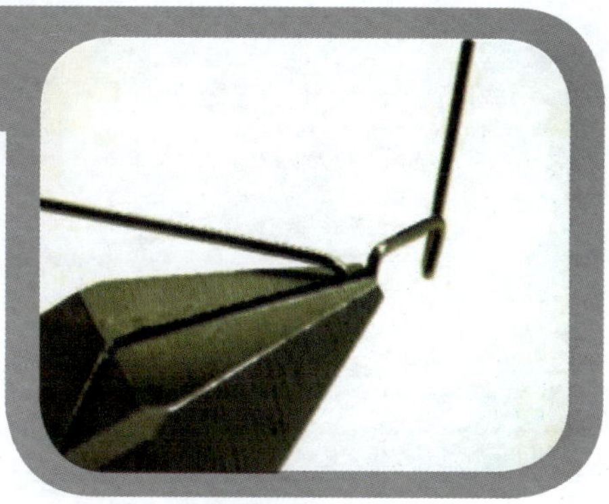

Second Bend From the Arrowhead. This Bend Should be Below the Height of the Bridge. This is Achieved by Clasping the Arrowhead Halfway up the Outer Side, Prior to Bending

15

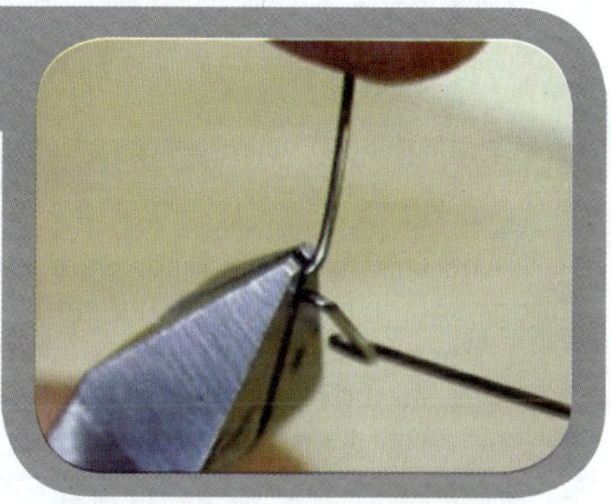

By Using the Tips of the Adam's Pliers, Adjust Bend Until Wire Touches Contact Point Prior to Crossing the Occlusion

16

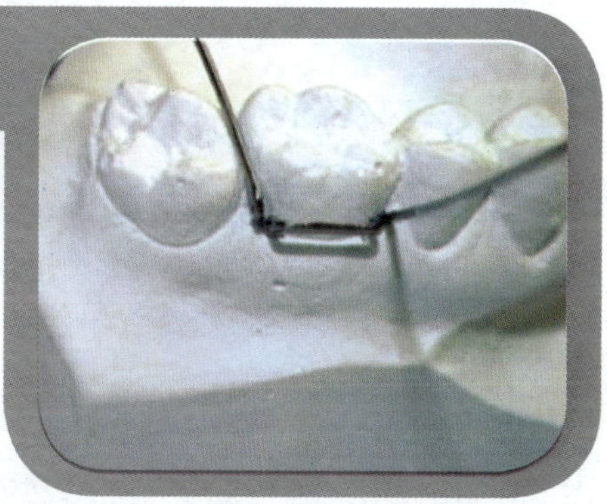

Check Position of Arrowheads and Angulations of Bridge. Angle of Bridge is 45° to Long Axis of Tooth

17

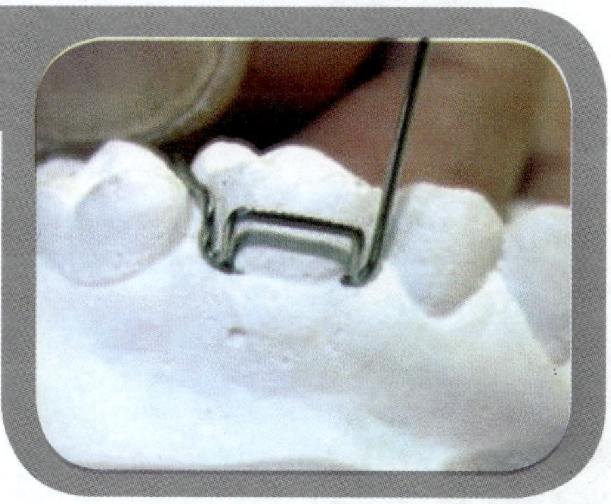

Adaptation of Wire Across Occlusion

18

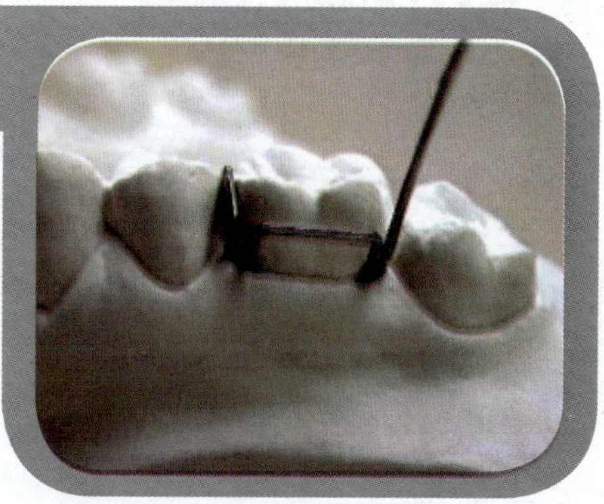

Check Position and Fit

19

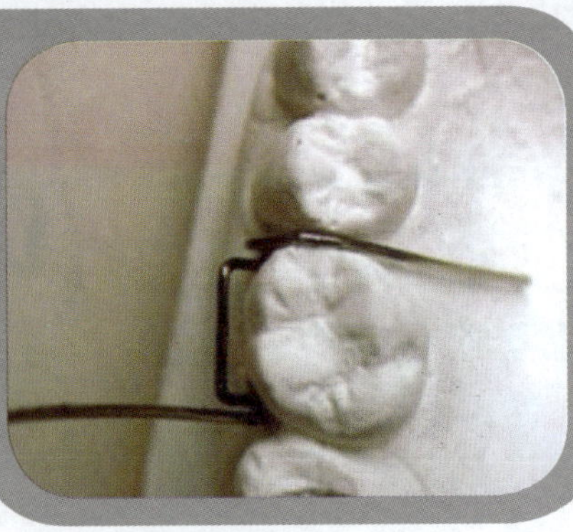

Bring Wire 2/3 into Palate to Form Tag End

20

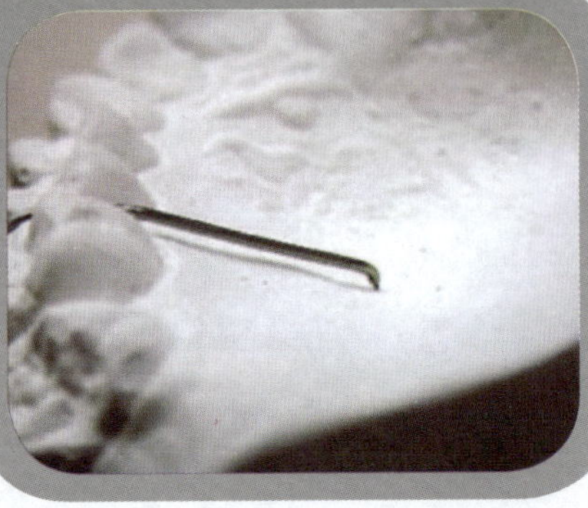

Uniform Spacing of 1mm With a Foot at the End of Tag

21

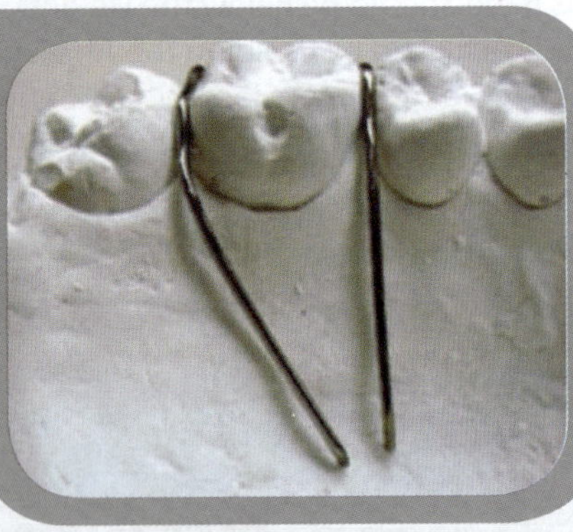

Distal Tagging Should Lie Forward to Allow Sufficient Space for Contour of Acrylic Baseplate

22

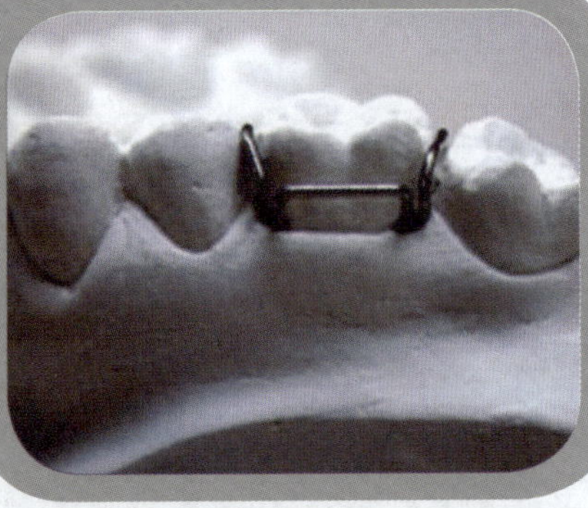

Arrowheads Must Engage Undercuts.
Bridge Should be of Sufficient Length to Allow Arrowheads to Engage Undercuts.
Bridge Should be Parallel to Occlusal Plane

23

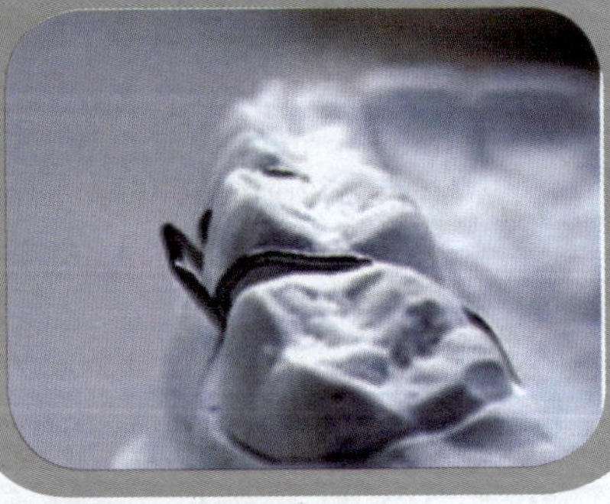

Bridge Should Lie at Approximately 45° to Long Axis of the Tooth

24

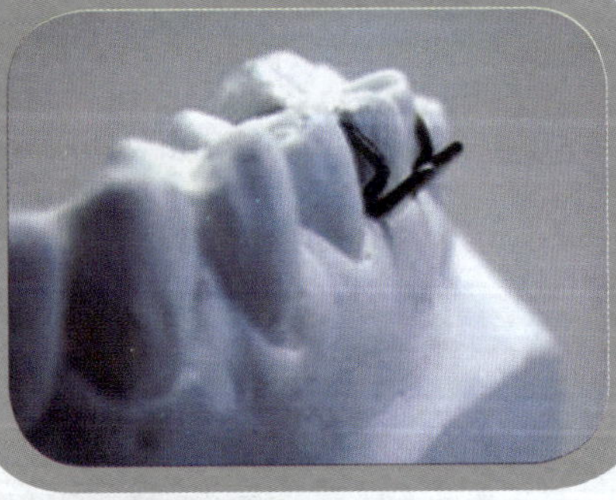

First Point of Contact out of the Arrowhead Should be the Contact Point Prior to Crossing the Occlusion

25

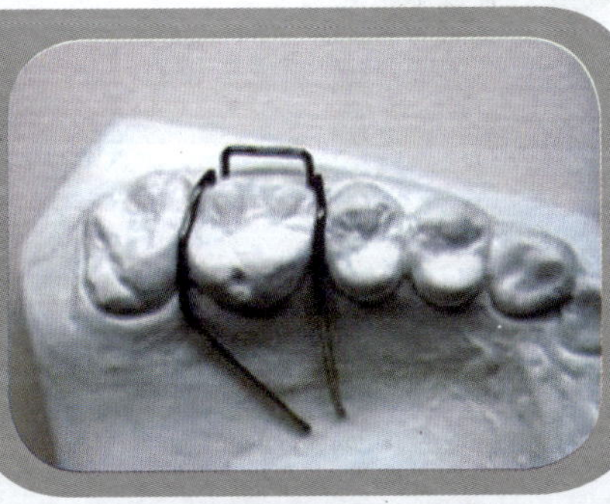

Adam's Clasp on Model

ADAM'S CLASP

Grading

Date : ____________________

Grade : ____________________

Sign : ____________________

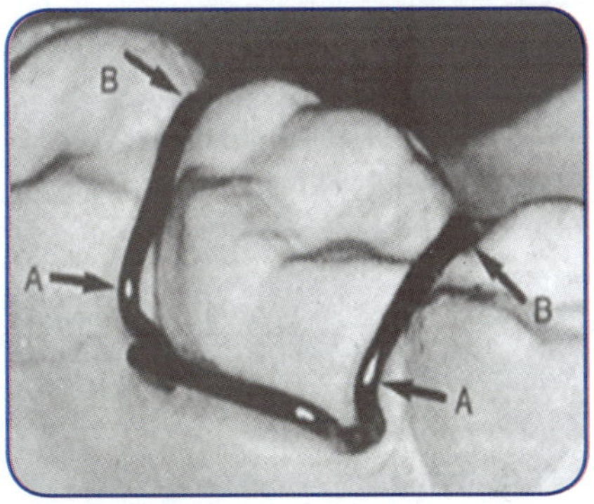

Close View of Adam's Clasp

Date : ____________________

Grade : ____________________

Sign : ____________________

Date : ____________________

Grade : ____________________

Sign : ____________________

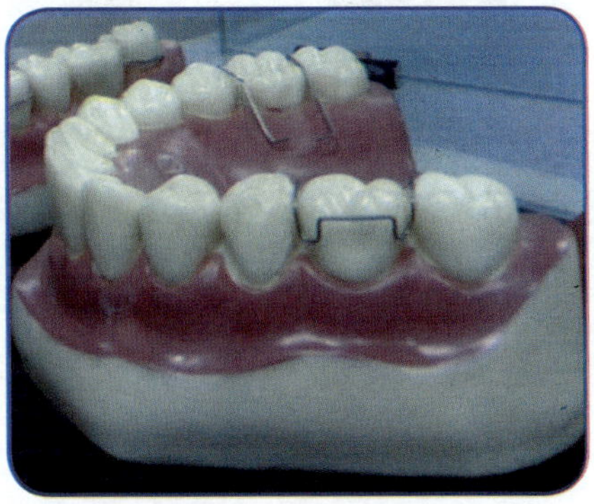

Adam's Clasp on Study Model

FABRICATION OF LABIAL BOW

STEPS OF LABIAL BOW

1

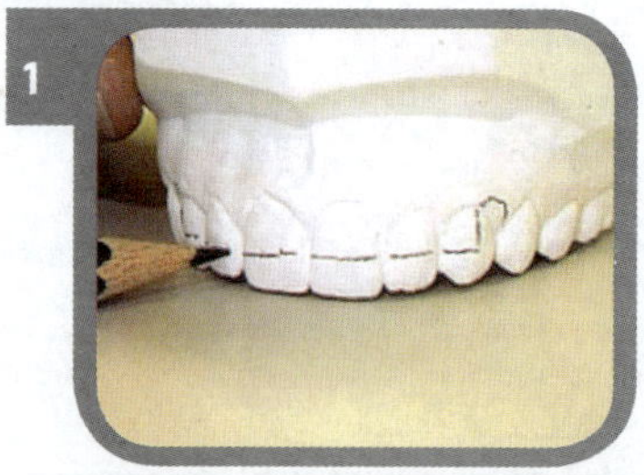

Draw a Line Mid Crown Height, Level With Occlusal Plane

2

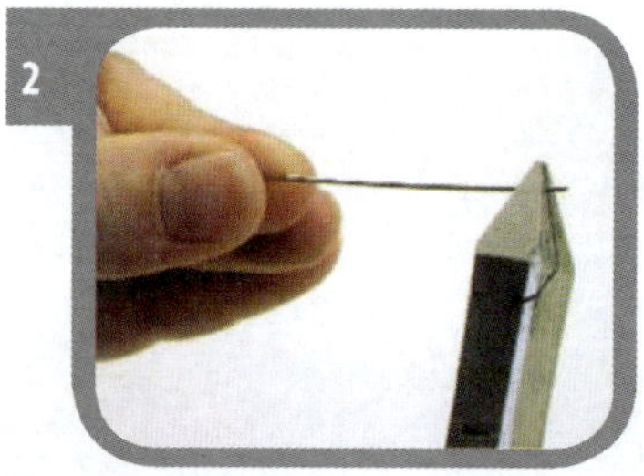

Cut a Length of 0.7mm Stainless Steel Wire, then Straighten Using Pliers and Fingers

3

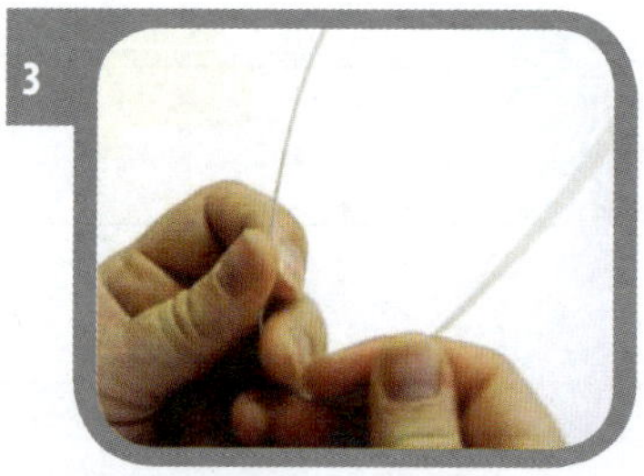

With Fingers and Thumbs, Form the Wire into an Ideal Arch

4

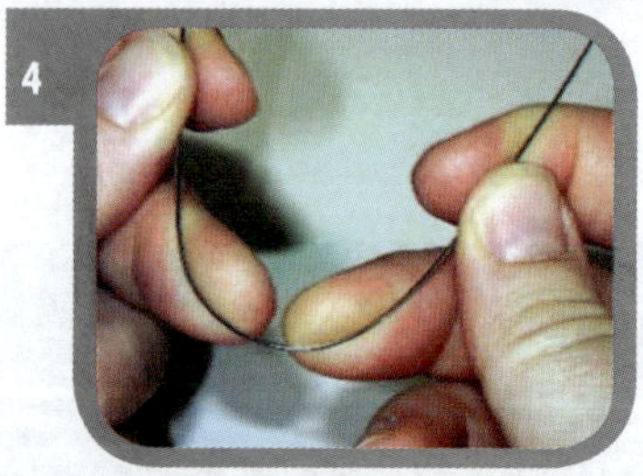

The Wire Will Bend in the Areas Where the Most Pressure is Applied

5

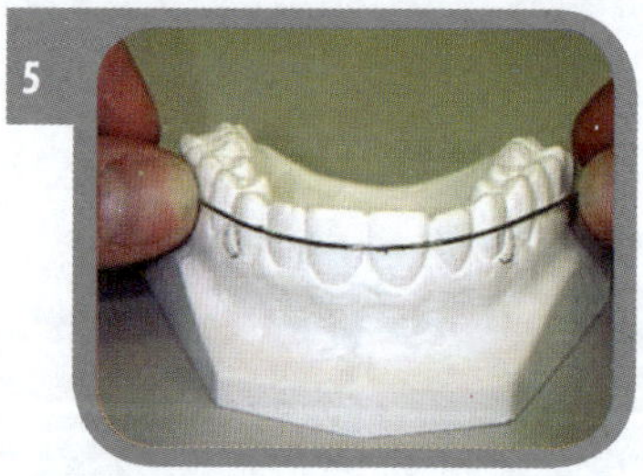

Try the Ideal Arch Against the Model, Using the Pencil Mark as a Guide. The Bow Should Rest Passively Against the Teeth

6

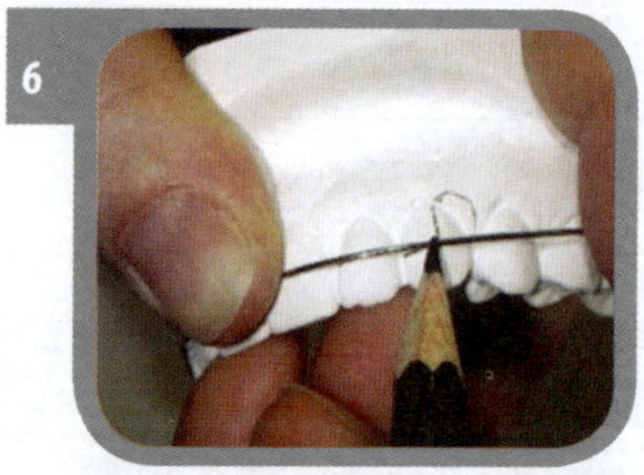

Using the Pencil Line as A Reference, Mark the Canine Eminence onto the Wire

7

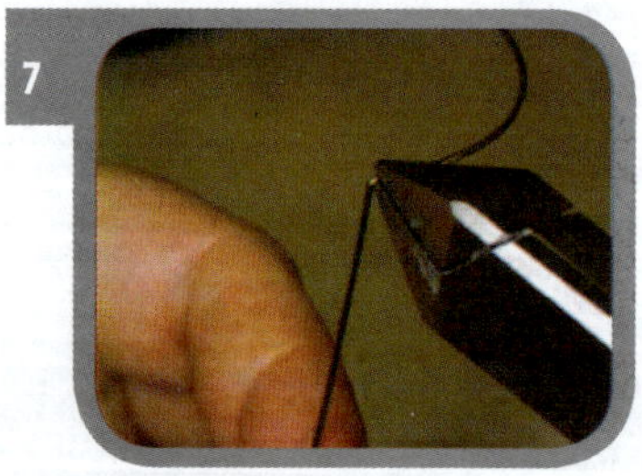

Make a 90° Bend

8

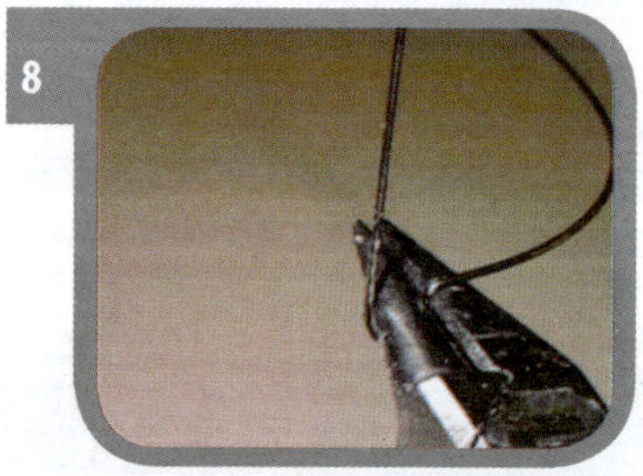

Using Spring Formers, Make a U-Loop. Length of U-Loop Should be Just Beyond Original Margin

9

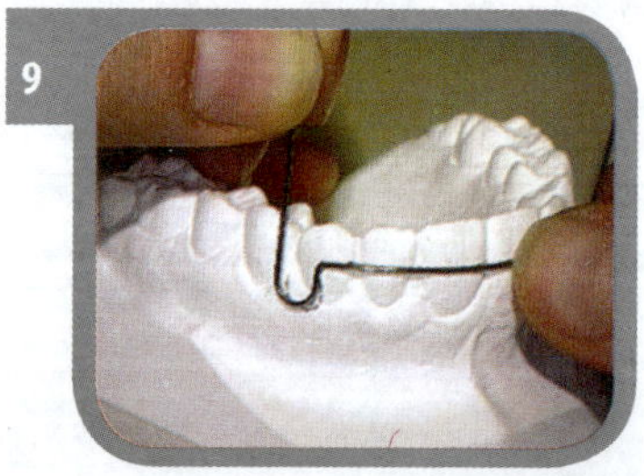

Check Against Model

10

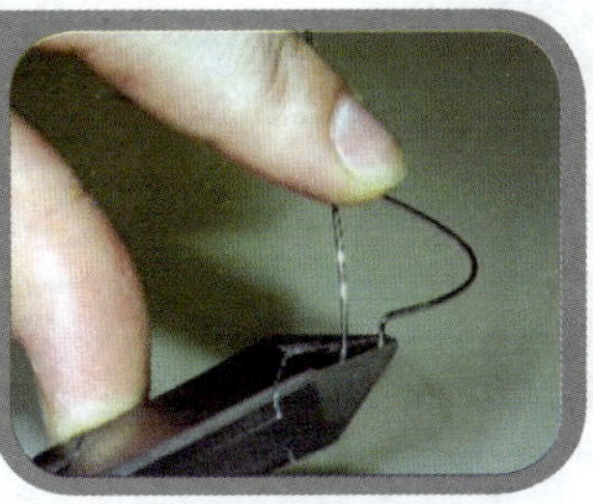

Contour Distal Section of U-Loop

11

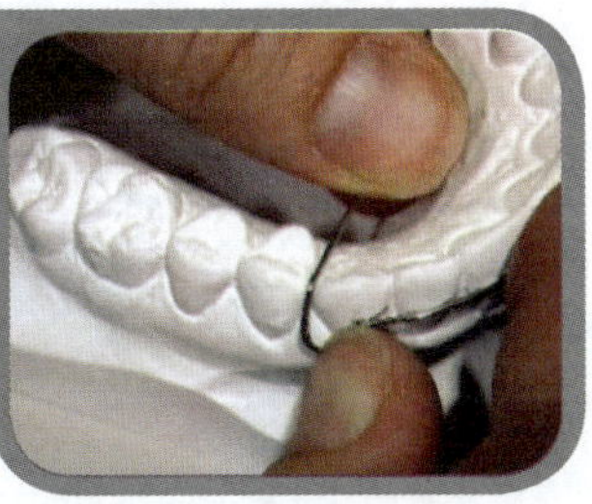

Bend Wire at Contact Point and Across Occlusion

12

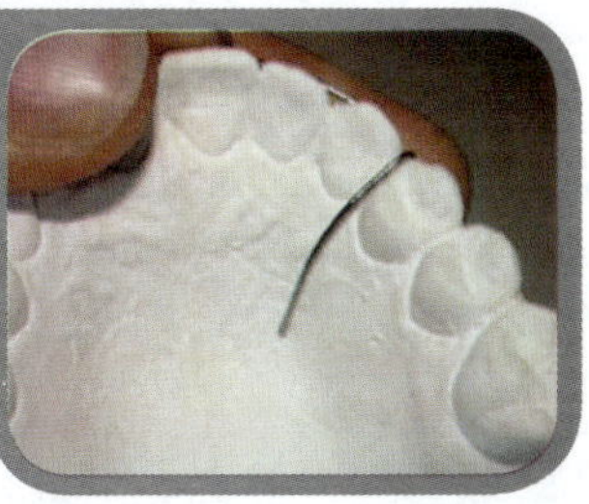

Tag End to Extend 2/3 into Palate

13

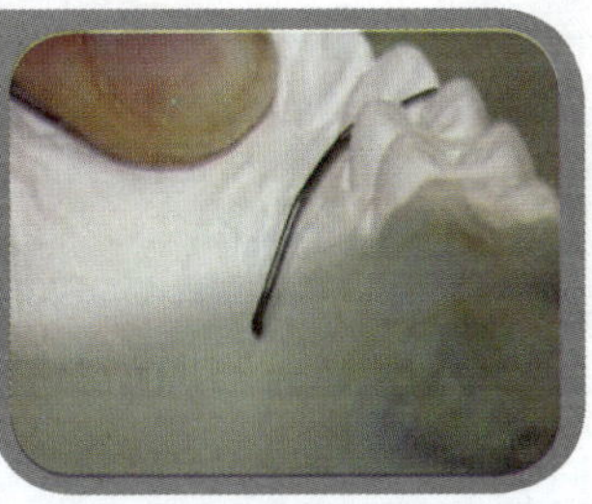

Uniform Spacing of 1mm, With a Foot at the End of Tag

14

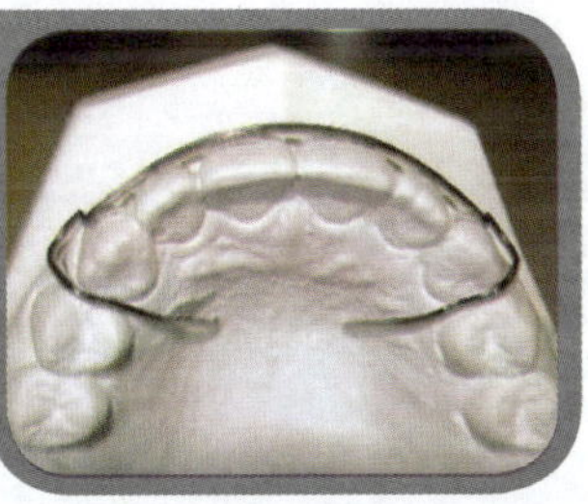

Occlusal View: Note that U-Loop Follows Contour of Arch

15

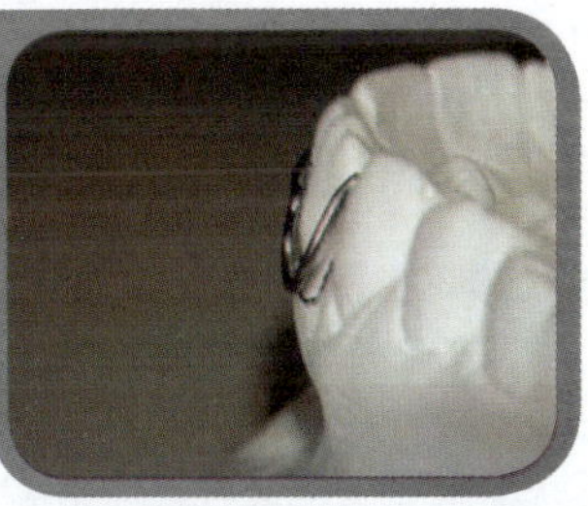

U-Loop Position Should Lie Approx. 1mm Away From Tissue

16

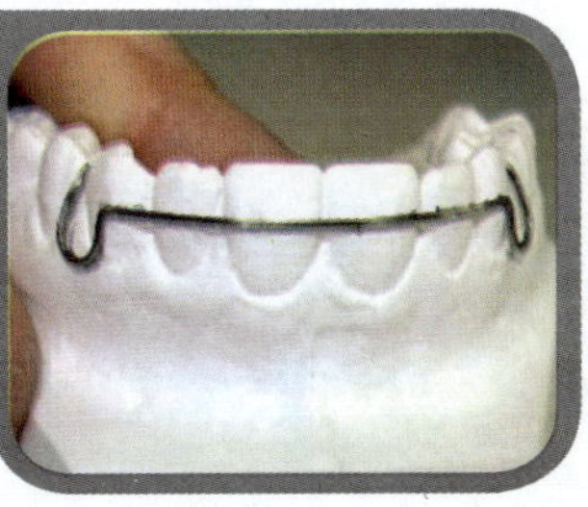

Labial Bow on Model

LABIAL BOW

Grading

Date : ____________________

Grade : ____________________

Sign : ____________________

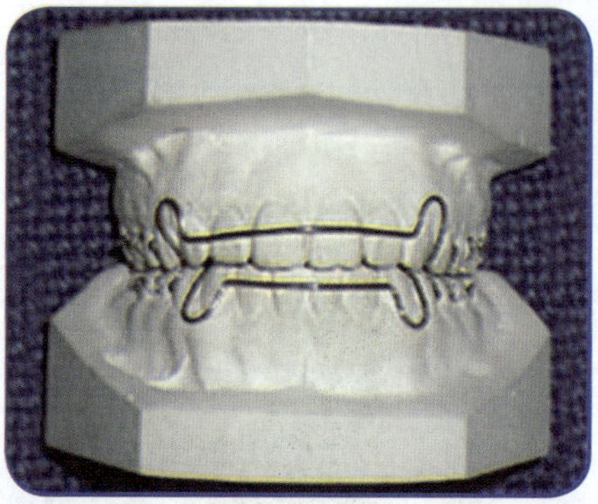

Frontal View of a Model

Date : ____________________

Grade : ____________________

Sign : ____________________

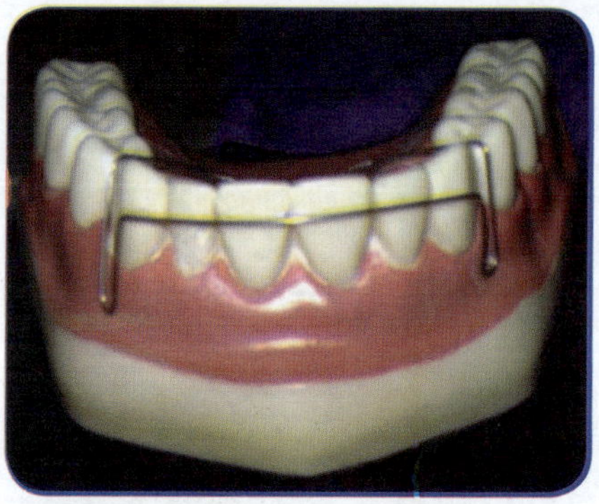

Labial View of Mandibular Jaw

Date : ____________________

Grade : ____________________

Sign : ____________________

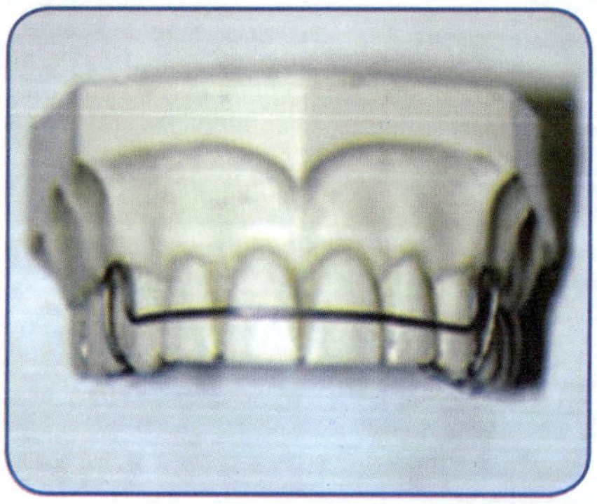

Labial View of Maxillary Jaw

ADAM'S CLASP AND LABIAL BOW IN ORTHODONTICS APPLIANCE (HAWLEYS RETAINER)

4
PRACTICAL

Grading

Date : ______________________

Grade : ______________________

Sign : ______________________

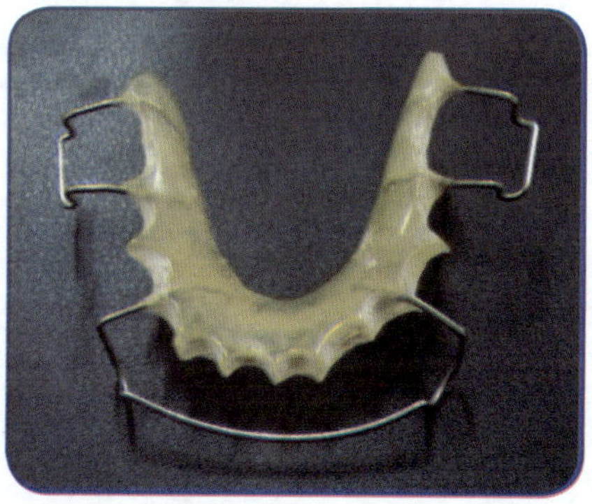

Hawleys Retainer

Date : ______________________

Grade : ______________________

Sign : ______________________

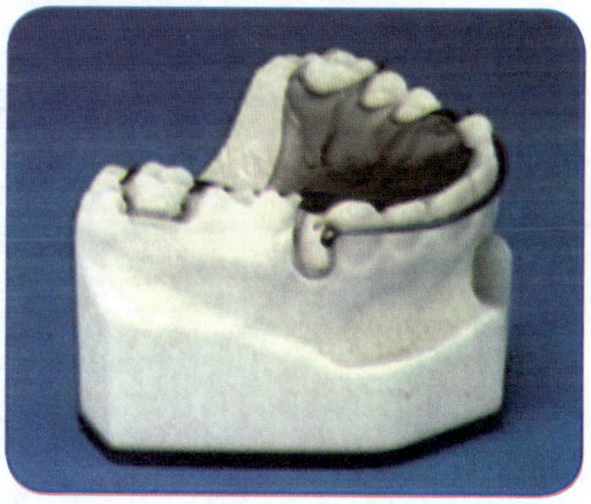

Hawleys Retainer on Model

5 PRACTICAL

FABRICATION OF T-SPRING

STEP 1

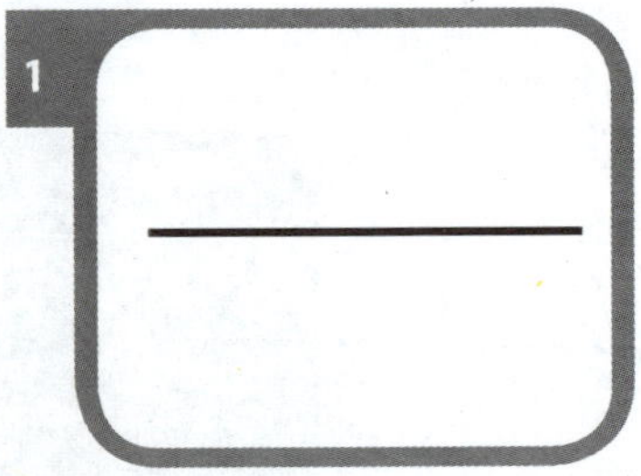

STEP 2

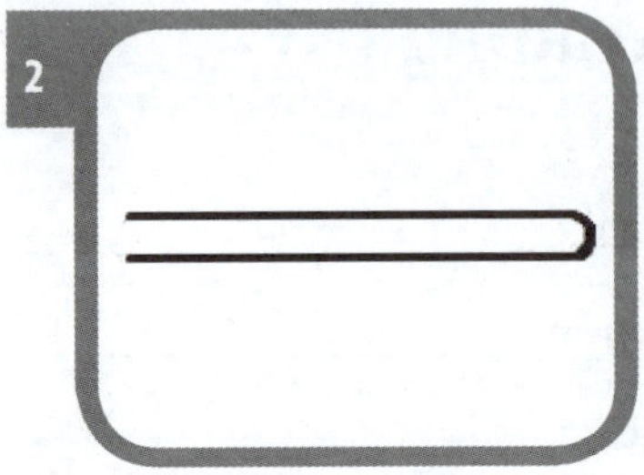

STEP 3

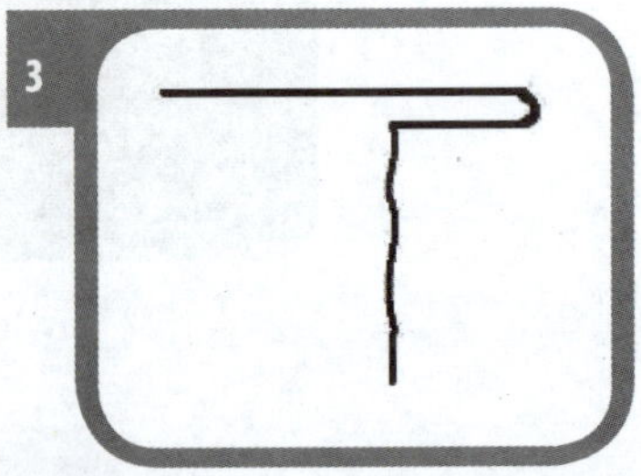

STEP 4

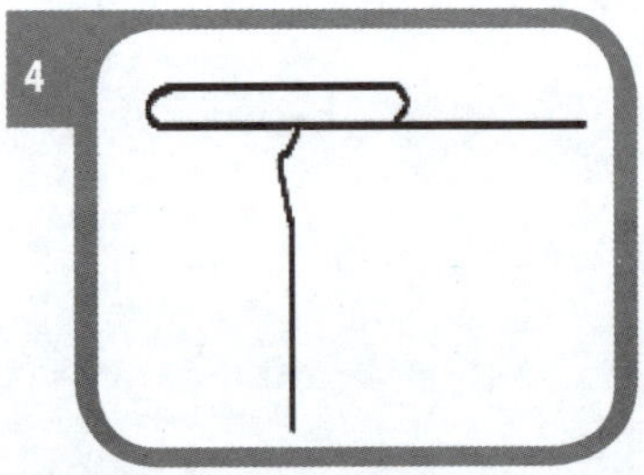

STEP 5

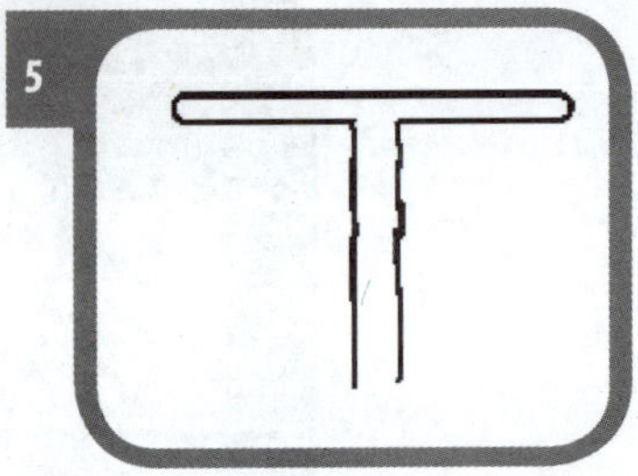

STEP 6

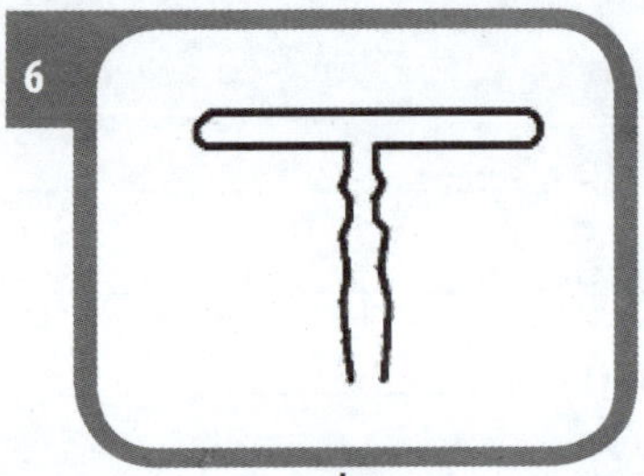

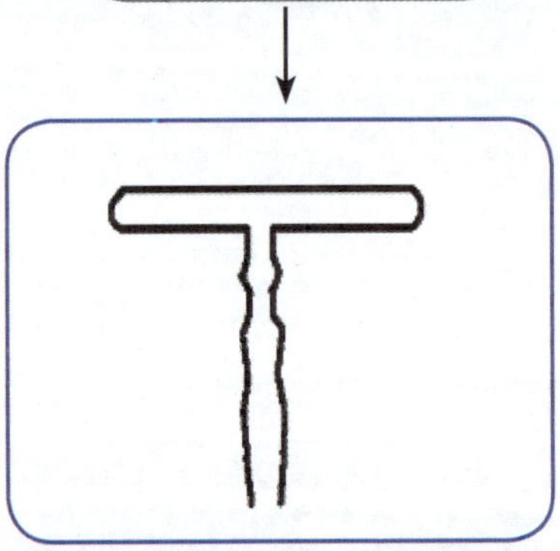

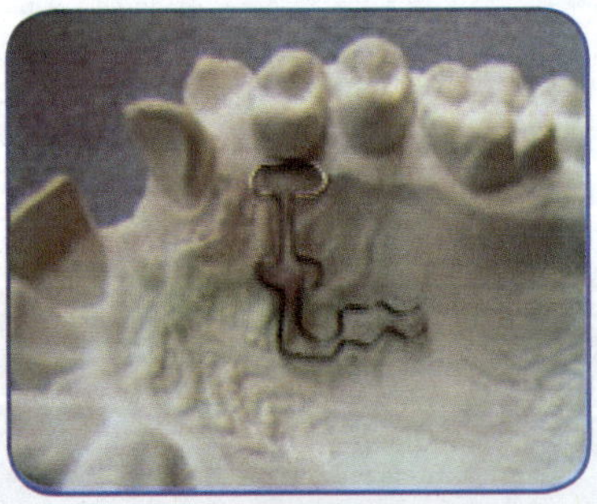

T-Spring on Model

T-SPRING

Grading

Date : ____________________

Grade : ____________________

Sign : ____________________

Date : ____________________

Grade : ____________________

Sign : ____________________

FABRICATION OF Z-SPRING (SPRING CANTILEVER)

6 PRACTICAL

STEP 1

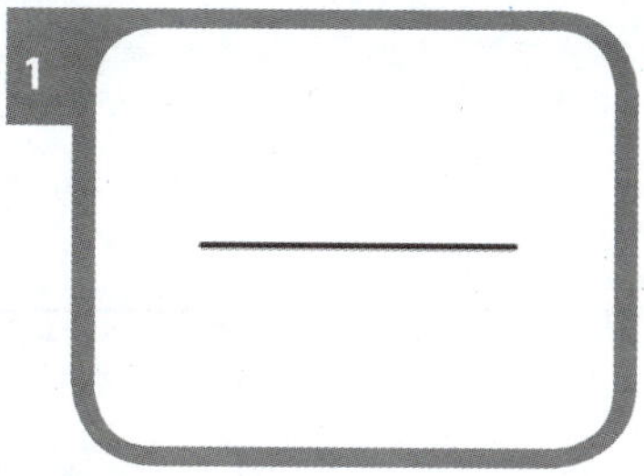

STEP 2

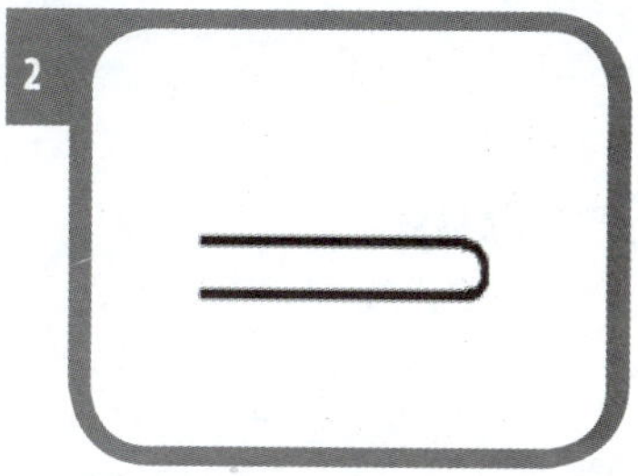

STEP 3

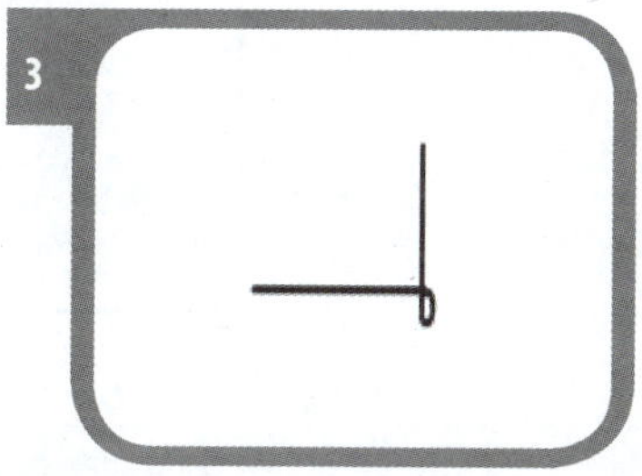

STEP 4

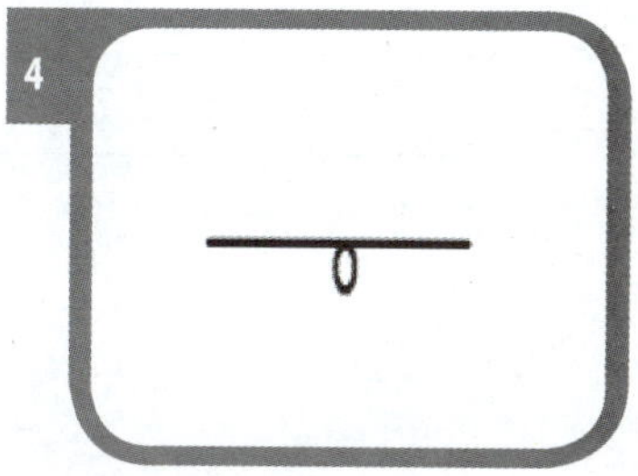

STEP 5

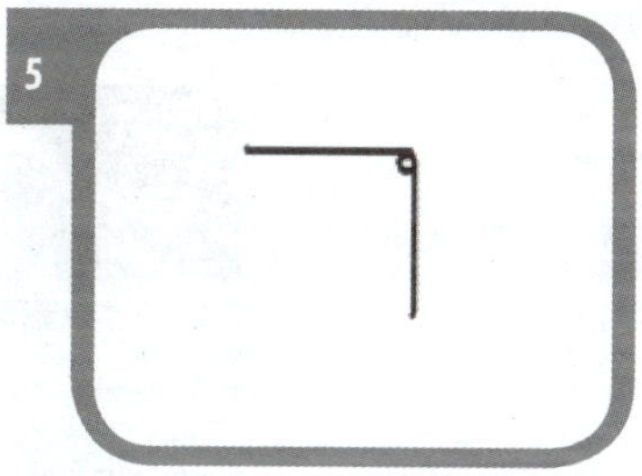

STEP 6

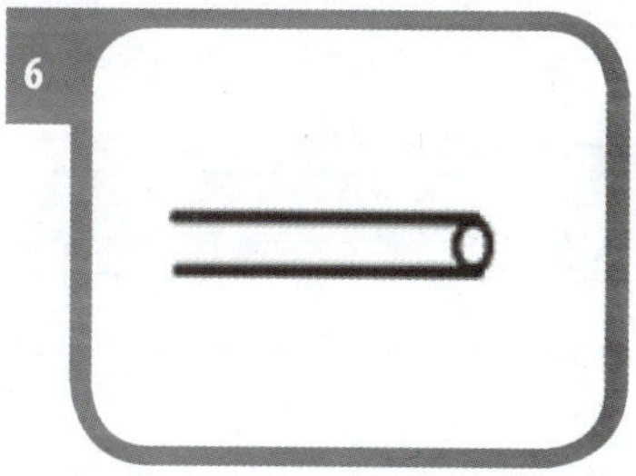

STEP 7

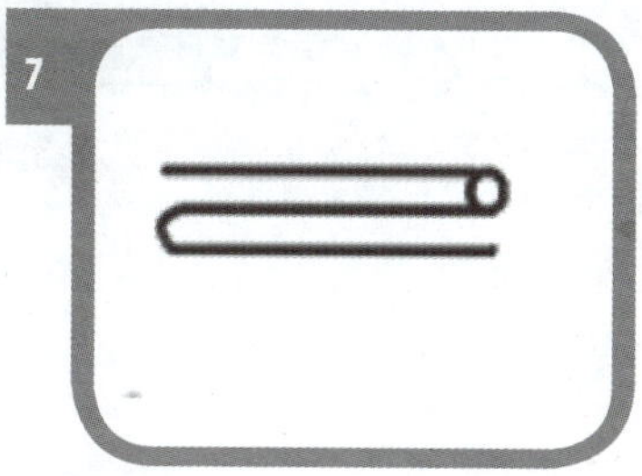

STEP 8

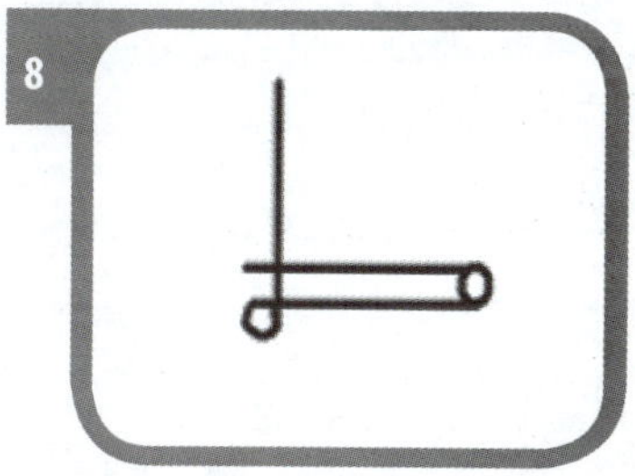

STEP 9

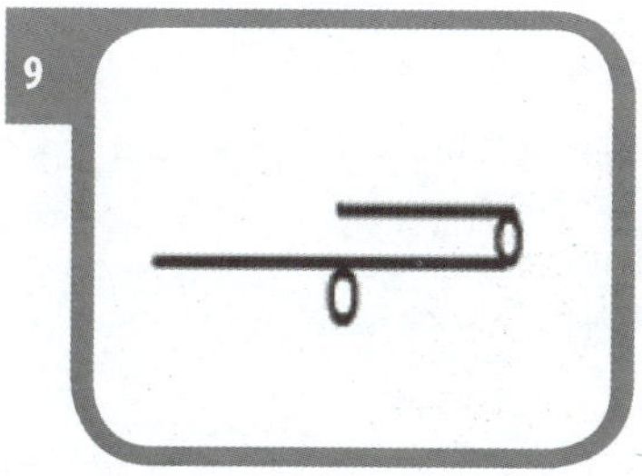

STEP 10

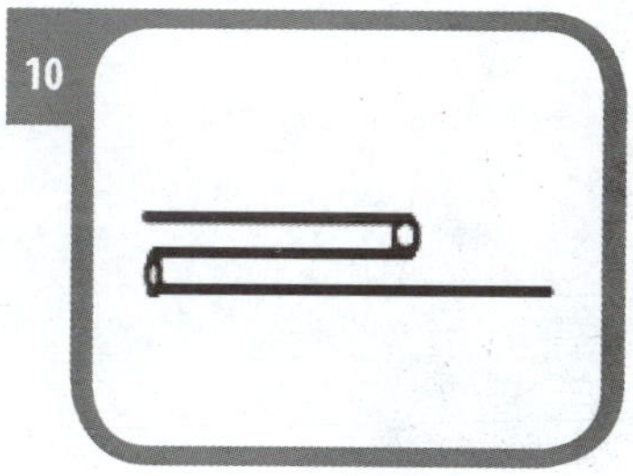

Z-SPRING

Grading

Date : ___________________________

Grade : ___________________________

Sign : ___________________________

Date : ___________________________

Grade : ___________________________

Sign : ___________________________

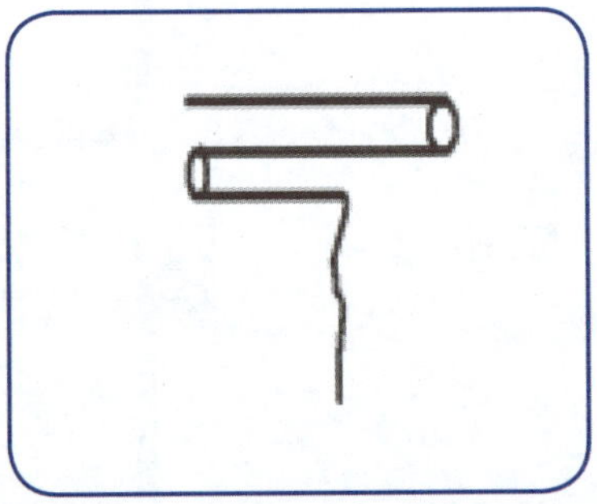

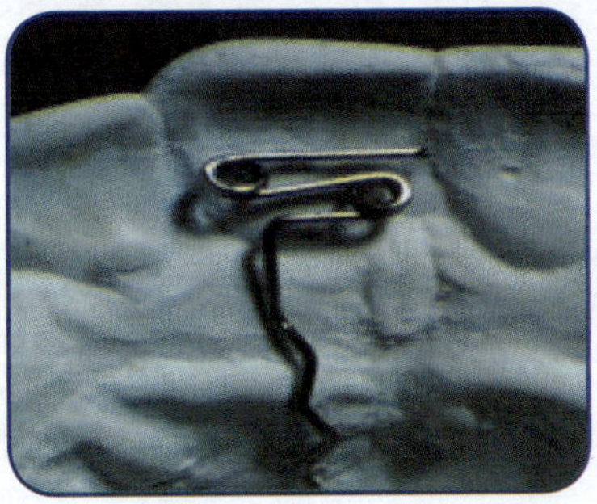

Z-Spring on Model

Grading

PREMOLAR (Right)

Date : ____________________

Grade : ____________________

Sign : ____________________

PREMOLAR (Left)

Date : ____________________

Grade : ____________________

Sign : ____________________

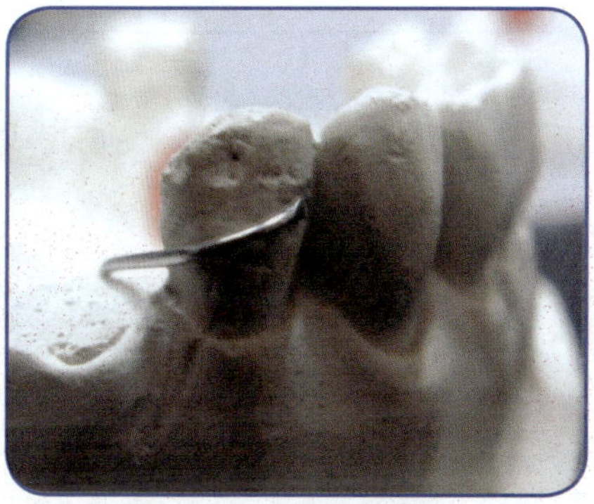

C-Clasp on Premolar

MOLAR (Right)

Date : ____________________

Grade : ____________________

Sign : ____________________

MOLAR (Left)

Date : ____________________

Grade : ____________________

Sign : ____________________

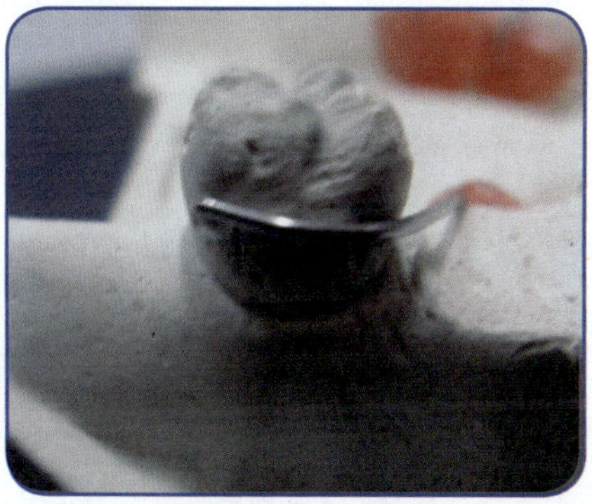

C-Clasp on Molar

8 PRACTICAL WAX UP AND SLAB MAKING

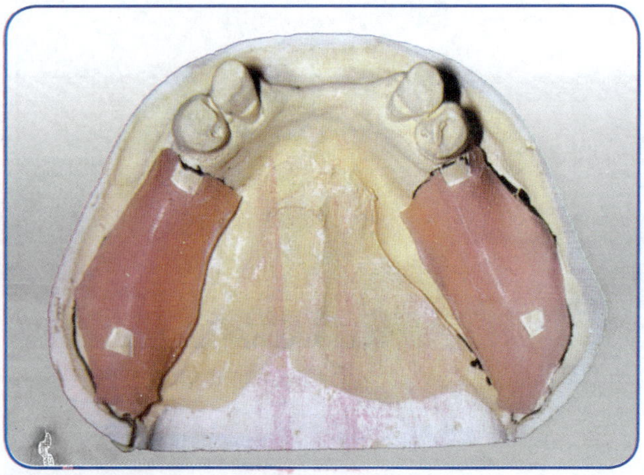

Wax up

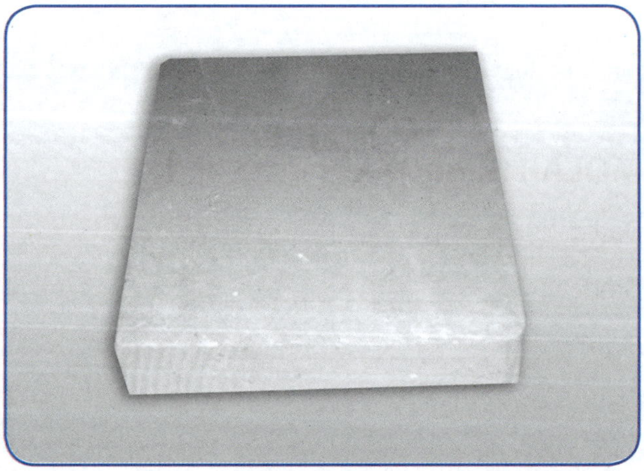

Plaster Slab

WAX UP

Grading

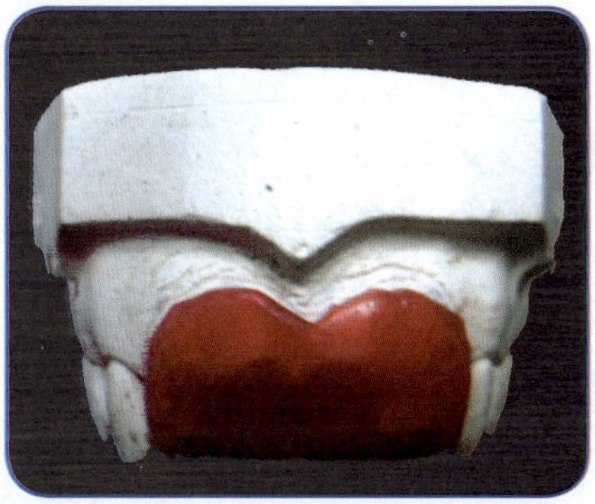
Frontal View of Maxillary Jaw

UPPER JAW

Date : ______________________

Grade : ______________________

Sign : ______________________

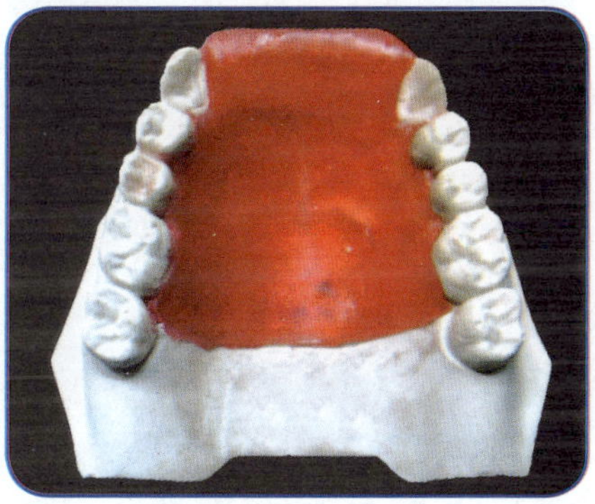
Palatal View of Maxillary Jaw

LOWER JAW

Right

Date : ______________________

Grade : ______________________

Sign : ______________________

Left

Date : ______________________

Grade : ______________________

Sign : ______________________

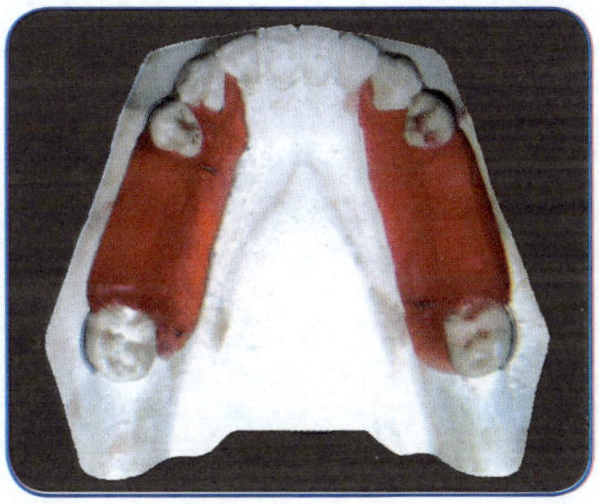
Occlusal View of Mandibular Jaw

Grading

Date : ____________________

Grade : ____________________

Sign : ____________________

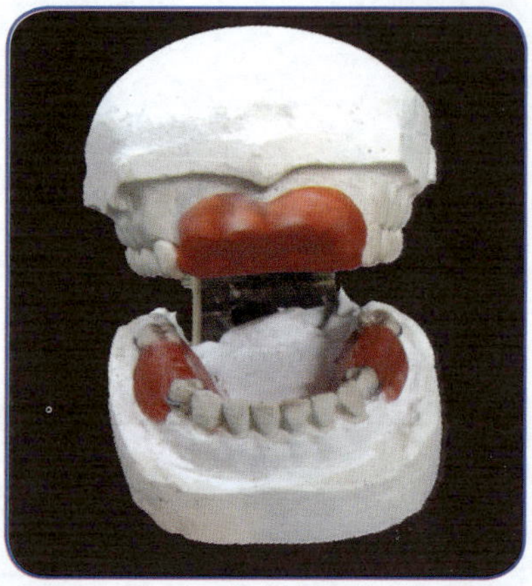

Frontal View

Date : ____________________

Grade : ____________________

Sign : ____________________

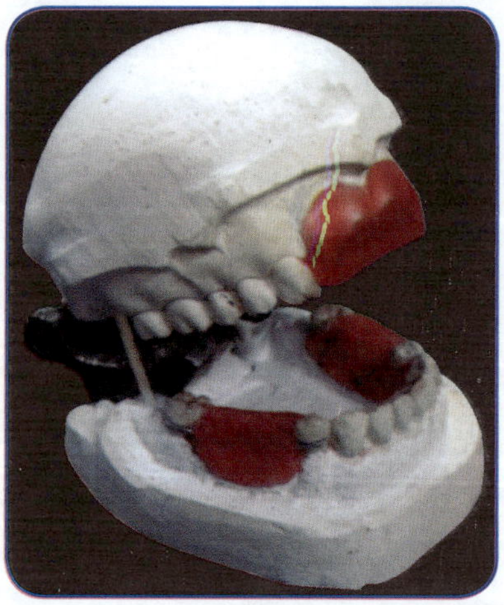

Lateral View

ARRANGEMENT OF TEETH

Grading

UPPER JAW

Date : ____________________

Grade : ____________________

Sign : ____________________

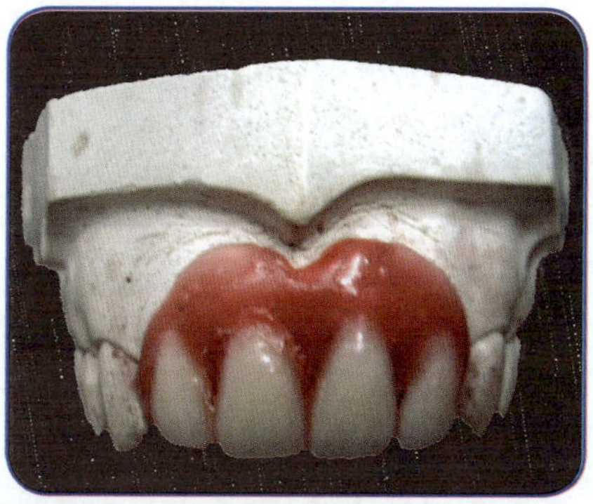

Labial View of Maxillary Jaw

LOWER JAW

Right

Date : ____________________

Grade : ____________________

Sign : ____________________

Left

Date : ____________________

Grade : ____________________

Sign : ____________________

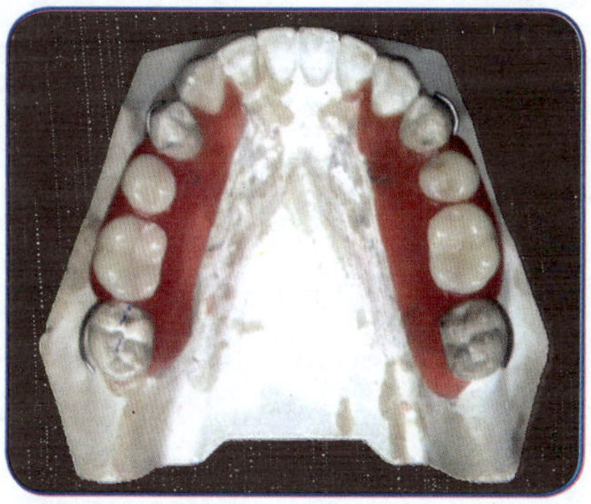

Occlusal View of Mandibular Jaw

SPECIFICATION FOR MIXING OF GYPSUM WITH WATER

MIXING RATIO OF DENTAL PLASTER AND WATER

Dental Plaster (Powder)		Water
2	:	1
300 gm	:	150 ml

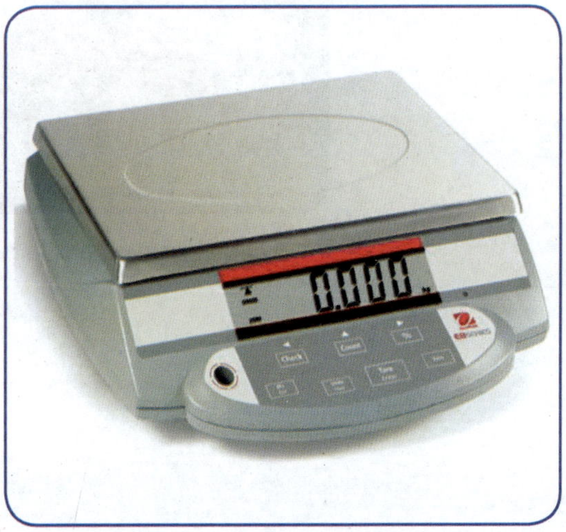

Weighing Balance for Measuring Powder

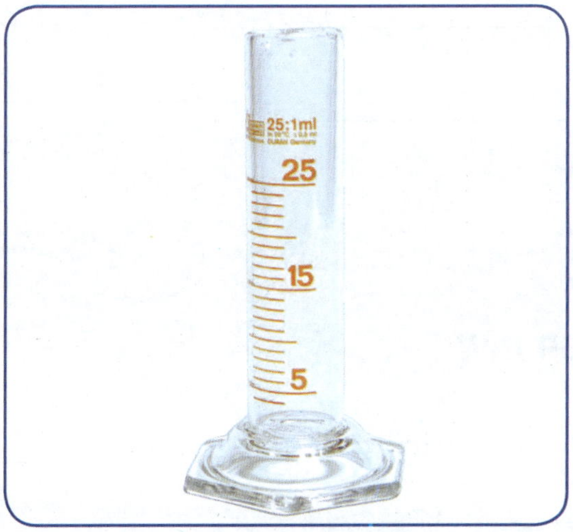

Glass Cylinder for Measuring Water

MIXING RATIO OF DENTAL STONE AND WATER

Dental Stone (Powder)		Water
3.5	:	1
350 gm	:	100 ml

MIXING GUIDE LINE OF GYPSUM WITH WATER

MIXING EQUIPMENT (MIXING BOWL AND SPATULA) SHOULD ALWAYS BE CLEAN AND FREE OF SET GYPSUM

STEP NO: 1

- Dispense measured room temperature water into mixing bowl

STEP NO: 2

- Add weighed gypsum slowly into water through the process of SIFTING

STEP NO: 3

- When all powder has been added into water allow it to soak for few seconds

  (This is an important step as it allows the gypsum to evenly hydrate without forming lumps)

STEP NO: 4

- Mixing of gypsum with water is done by curved ended spatula
- Mixing begins with a unicircular motion and incorporates all the powder particles
- Wipe the blade of spatula against the side and bottom of mixing bowl to ensure that all the powder is being wetted
- The consistency of the final mix should be that of creamy and lump free

STEP NO:5

- Vibrate or tap the mixing bowl to remove air bubbles that might have formed during mixing

DONTS

- Spatulation for longer duration
- Spatulation too vigorously
- Change powder/water ratio during mixing
- Add freshly gypsum over a partially hardened mixture
- Stir the mixture too long as it will start to harden
- Drop gypsum handsfuls directly into water

PLASTER SLAB/PLASTER BLOCK

PLASTER SLAB

Grading

Date : ______________________

Grade : ______________________

Sign : ______________________

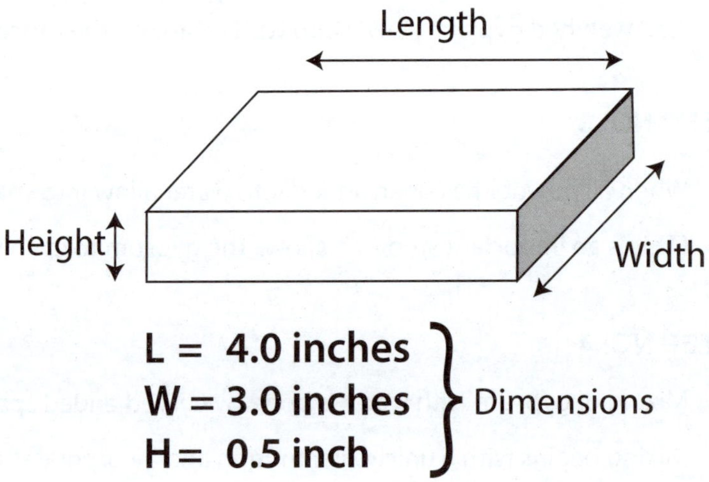

Date : ______________________

Grade : ______________________

Sign : ______________________

PLASTER BLOCK

Grading

Date : ______________________

Grade : ______________________

Sign : ______________________

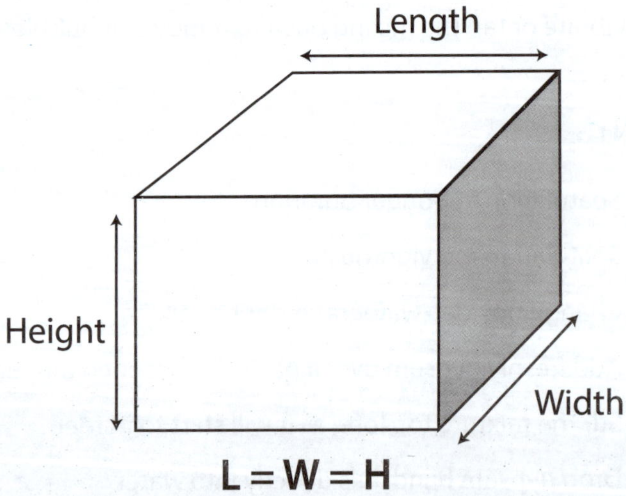

Date : ______________________

Grade : ______________________

Sign : ______________________

TRIMMING AND FINISHING STUDY MODELS

Student Name:____________________________ **Date:**__________________________

TRIMMING AND FINISHING STUDY MODELS

STUDENT		STUDY MODELS		FACULTY
MAX	MAND		MAX	MAND
		OVER ALL		
		1. All teeth and anatomy are preserved (none removed through trimming; no broken or chipped teeth)		
		2. Stone is smooth; no voids or blebs> 1 mm; cleared of dust and trimming debris		
		BASES		
		3. Occluded models and occlusal plane are parallel to the benchtop (height does not differ by >1/8 inch)		
		4. Bases are smooth and flat; no bevels; does not rock (a nail file will not slide under)		
		5. Height of occluded models is 2.5 to 2.75 inches.		
		6. Bases are 1/3 of height; anatomy is 2/3 of height in anterior region		
		BORDERS		
		7. Posterior borders are flat and bite will not open when occluded models are placed on their backs (<1mm)		
		8. Arch length extends atleast 0.25 inch beyond most posterior teeth, not removing maxillary tuberosity, hamular notch or mandibular retromolar areas		
		9. Back of maxillary model is perpendicular to median line <30		
		10. The vestibule is not removed by trimming		
		11. Sides are flush, flat and smooth		
		OTHERS		
		12. Tongue area is flat and smooth without removing any anatomy		
		13. Models are labeled with students or patients name and date		

Laboratory: #____________ criteria must be performed satisfactorily

Instructor Remarks: ____

ARMAMENTARIUM USED FOR TRIMMING AND FINISHING THE MODELS

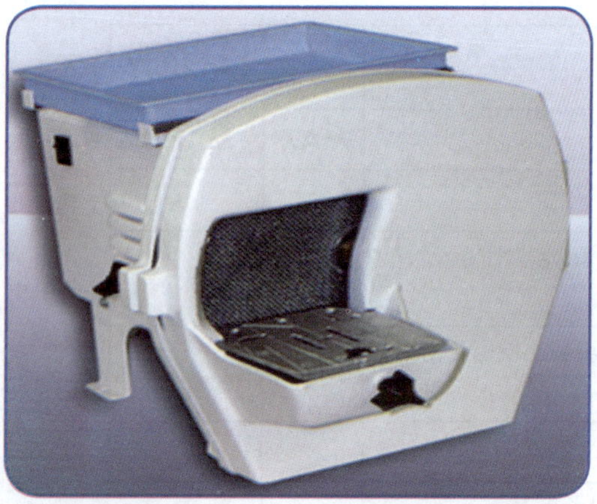

Model Trimmer

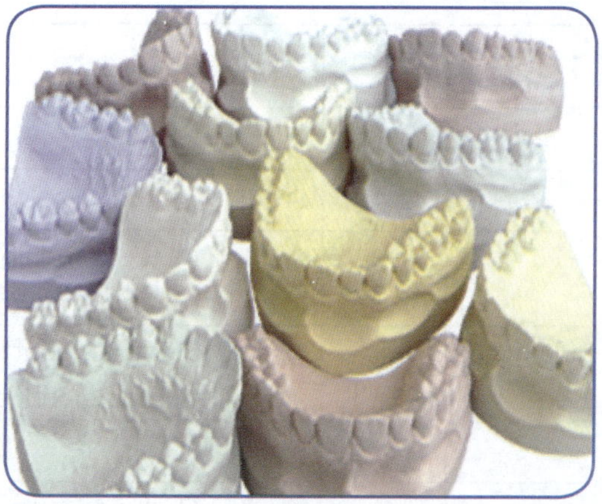

Gypsum Model

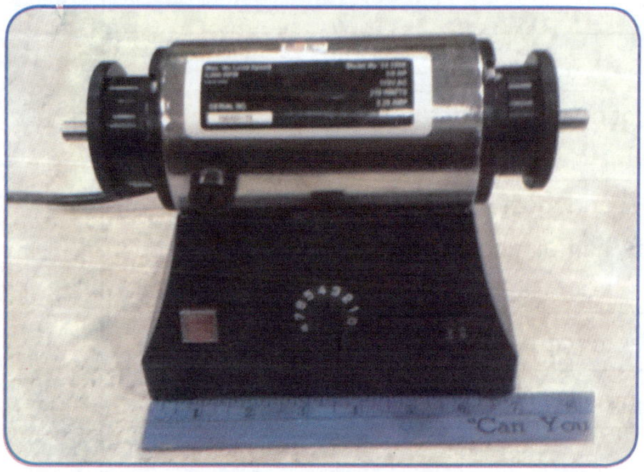

Grinder

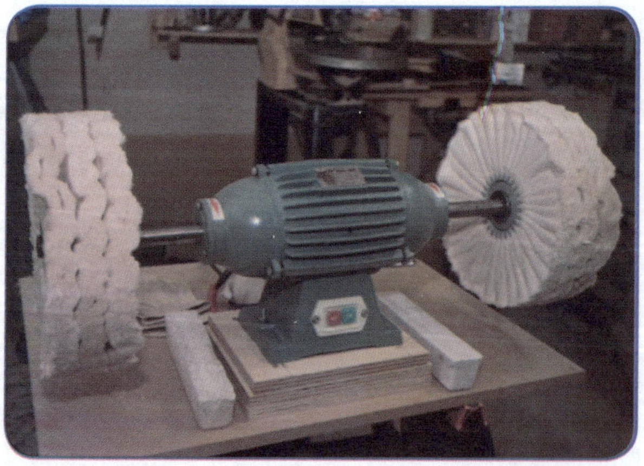

Buffing Machine

Section B

9

PRACTICAL

MANIPULATION OF DENTAL CEMENTS

Student Name:____________________________ **Date:**__________________________

MIXING ZINC PHOSPHATE CEMENT FOR LUTING AND AS A BASE

Satisfactory performance of this lab/clinical skill is expected. The student is to self evaluate the designated column. After faculty evaluation, the skill performance is to be discussed based on both evaluations.

If satisfactory, the skill evaluation is complete. If unsatisfactory, remediation will occur until criteria is performed satisfactorily.

CRITERIA	INSTRUCTOR		STUDENT	
1: Luting Consistency	**S**	**U**	**S**	**U**
Powder is properly incorporated into the liquid				
Mix is completed within the specified mixing time				
Mix will form a "1 inch string" between the spatula and slab				
2: Base Consistency				
Powder is properly incorporated into the liquid				
Mix is completed within specified mixing time				
Mix is thick, putty like, and shaped into a ball				

Faculty please identify minimum lab and clinical competency levels:

Laboratory: #______________ criteria must be performed satisfactorily

Clinical: #______________ criteria must be performed satisfactorily

Time Started: __________________ Time Completed: __________________

Instructor Remarks: ____

Suggestions/Comments:

____

____

____

____

S= Satisfactory U= Unsatisfactory

Note:

Follow the mixing instruction according to page # 38-40

ARMAMENTARIUM FOR MIXING ZINC PHOSPHATE CEMENT
Zinc phosphate powder
Zinc phosphate liquid
Cement spatula
Powder scoop
Glass slab

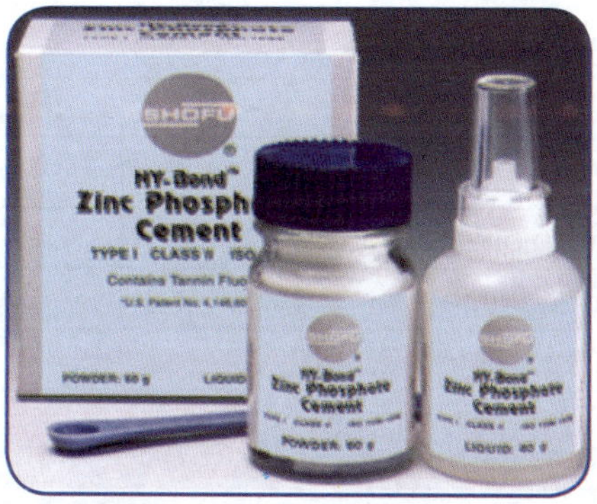

Zinc Phosphate Powder and Liquid

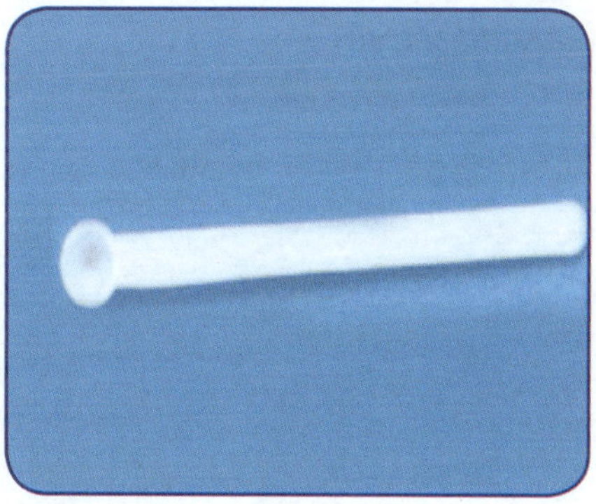
Scoop

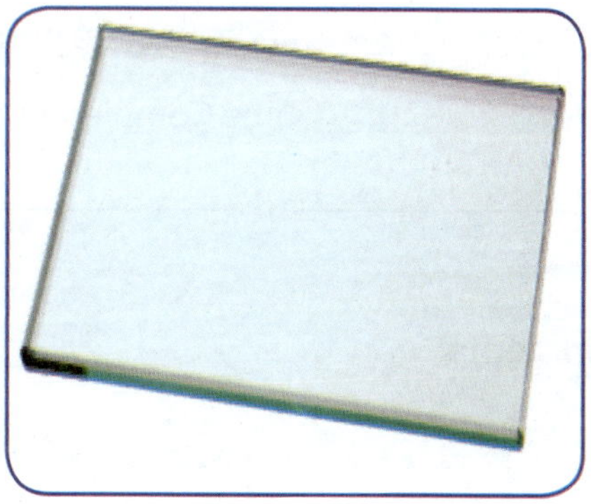
Glass Slab

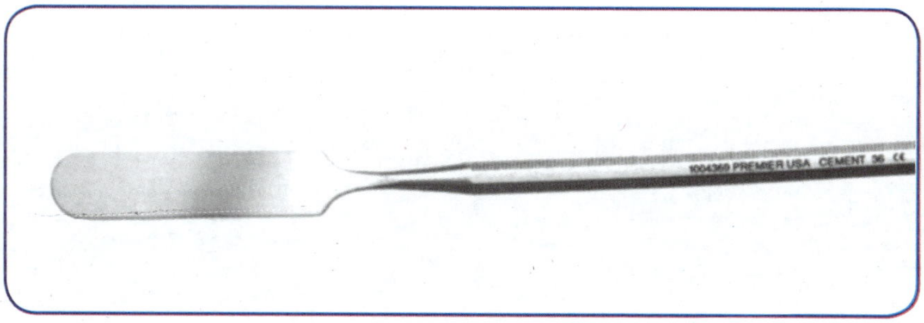
Cement Spatula

Student Name:____________________ **Date:**____________________

MIXING GLASS IONOMER CEMENT – LUTING CONSISTENCY

Satisfactory performance of this lab/clinical skill is expected. The student is to self evaluate the designated column. After faculty evaluation, the skill performance is to be discussed based on both evaluations.

If satisfactory, the skill evaluation is complete. If unsatisfactory, remediation will occur until criteria is performed satisfactorily.

CRITERIA	INSTRUCTOR		STUDENT	
	S	U	S	U
1. The powder is incorporated into liquid in one portion				
2. The mix is completed within the specified time				
3. The completed mix will stretch at least a half inch				

Faculty please identify minimum lab and clinical competency levels:

Laboratory: #____________ criteria must be performed satisfactorily

Clinical: #____________ criteria must be performed satisfactorily

Time Started: ____________ Time Completed: ____________

Instructor Remarks: ________________________

Suggestions/Comments:

____

____

____

____

Note:

Follow the mixing instruction according to page # 38-40

ARMAMENTARIUM FOR MIXING GLASS IONOMER CEMENT
Glass ionomer powder
Glass ionomer liquid
Dispensing scoop
Cement spatula
Glass slab

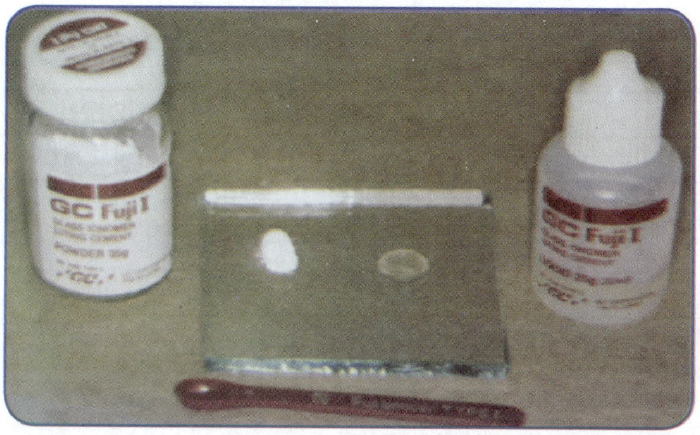

Glass Ionomer Powder, Liquid, Scoop and Glass Slab

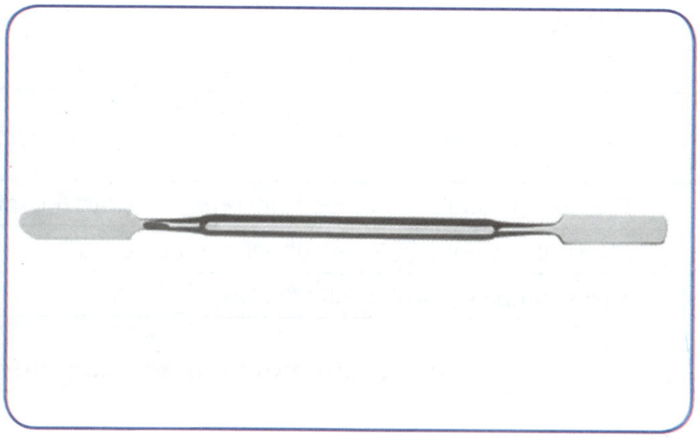

Cement Spatula

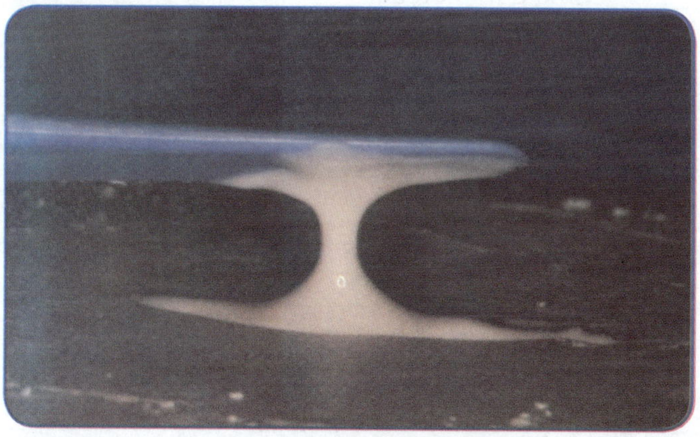

Proper Luting Consistency of Glass Ionomer Cement

Student Name:____________________ **Date:**____________________

MIXING ZINC OXIDE EUGENOL AS A BASE OR TEMPORARY RESTORATIVE MATERIAL

Satisfactory performance of this lab/clinical skill is expected. The student is to self evaluate the designated column. After faculty evaluation, the skill performance is to be discussed based on both evaluations.

If satisfactory, the skill evaluation is complete. If unsatisfactory, remediation will occur until criteria is performed satisfactorily.

CRITERIA	INSTRUCTOR		STUDENT	
	S	U	S	U
1. Powder and liquid are properly incorporated into the mix				
2. Mix is consistent and has a putty like appearence				
3. Mix is completed within 1.5 minutes				

Faculty please identify minimum lab and clinical competency levels:

Laboratory: #______________ criteria must be performed satisfactorily

Clinical : #______________ criteria must be performed satisfactorily

Time Started: ________________ Time Completed: ________________

Instructor Remarks: ____________________________________

Suggestions/Comments:

____

____

____

____

Note:

Follow the mixing instruction according to page # 38-40

ARMAMENTARIUM FOR MIXING ZINC OXIDE EUGENOL CEMENT
Zinc oxide powder
Cement spatula
Eugenol liquid
Glass slab
Dropper

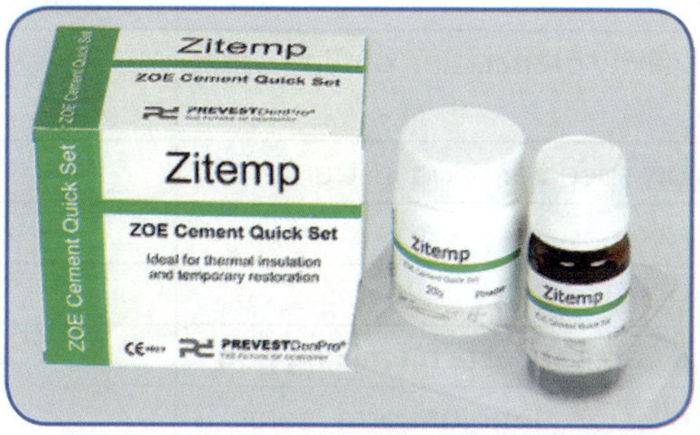

Zinc Oxide Eugenol Powder and Liquid

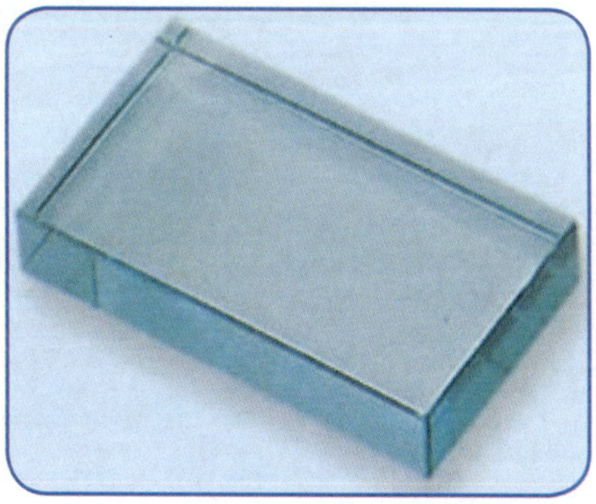

Glass Slab

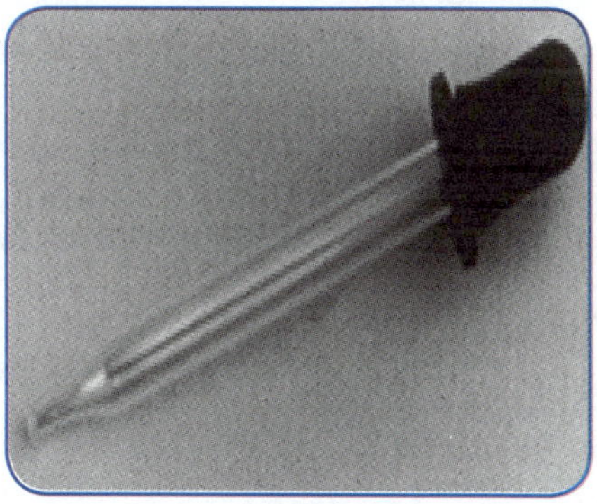

Dropper

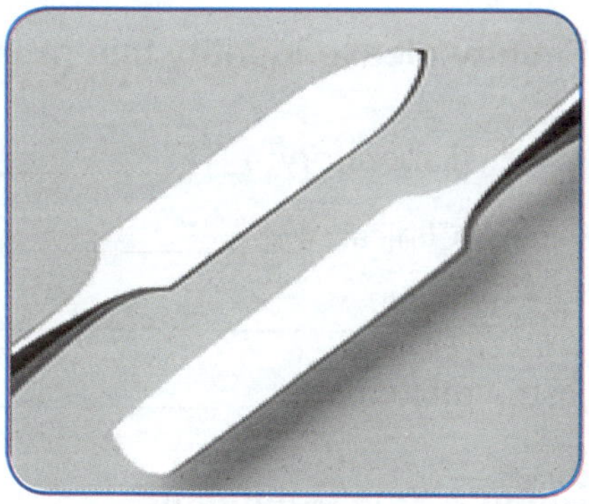

Cement Spatula

Student Name:____________________ **Date:**________________

MIXING CALCIUM HYDROXIDE FOR CAVITY LINING

Satisfactory performance of this lab/clinical skill is expected. The student is to self evaluate the designated column. After faculty evaluation, the skill performance is to be discussed based on both evaluations.

If satisfactory, the skill evaluation is complete. If unsatisfactory, remediation will occur until criteria is performed satisfactorily.

CRITERIA	INSTRUCTOR		STUDENT	
	S	U	S	U
1. Isolate with rubber dam, complete cavity preparation outline using high speed burs				
2. Excavate caries (if present) using slow speed or hand instruments				
3. Rinse cavity with 2.6% - 5% NaoCl				
4. Dry preparation with cotton pellet				
5. Dispence equal volume of Base and Catalyst paste on mixing pad				
6. Stir immediately with Dycal applicator until uniform color is achieved				
7. Mixing is done within 10 seconds				
8. Using dycal liner applicator, place the mix on exposed pulp (thickness should be less than 1mm)				

Faculty please identify minimum lab and clinical competency levels:

Laboratory: #__________ criteria must be performed satisfactorily

Clinical : #__________ criteria must be performed satisfactorily

Time Started: __________ Time Completed: __________

Instructor Remarks: ____________________

Suggestions/Comments:

ARMAMENTARIUM FOR CALCIUM HYDROXIDE CEMENT
Calcium hydroxide (Base and Catalyst)
Mixing paper pad
Dycal applicator

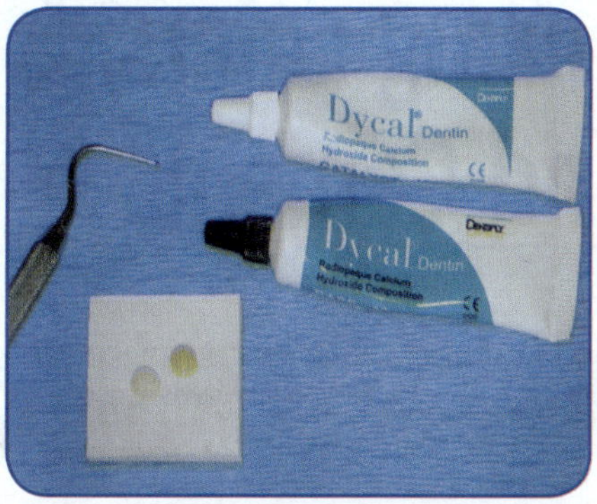

Calcium Hydroxide Dispensed on
Mixing Paper Pad

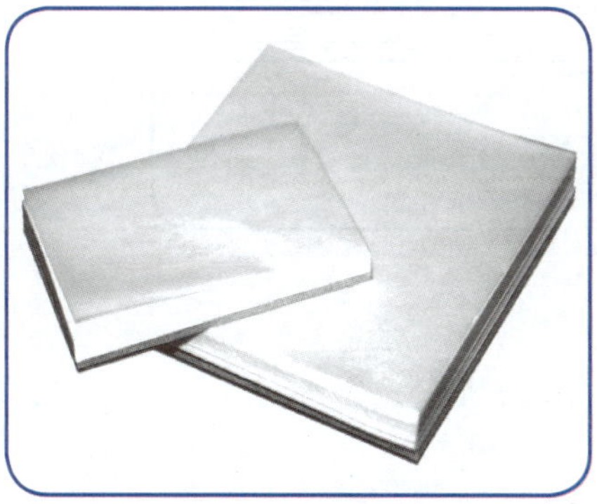
Mixing Pad

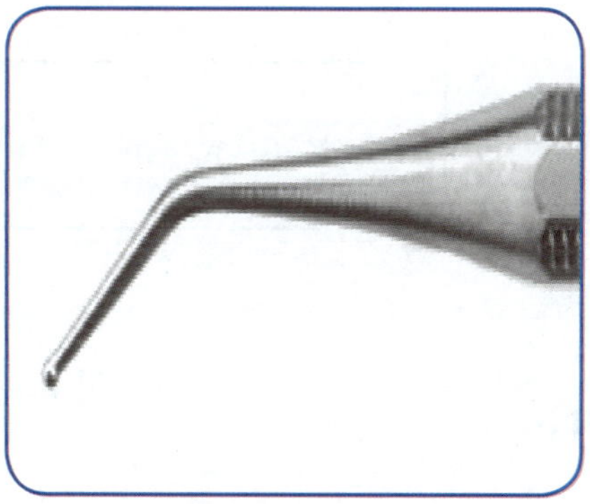
Dycal Applicator

MIXING OF POWDER AND LIQUID

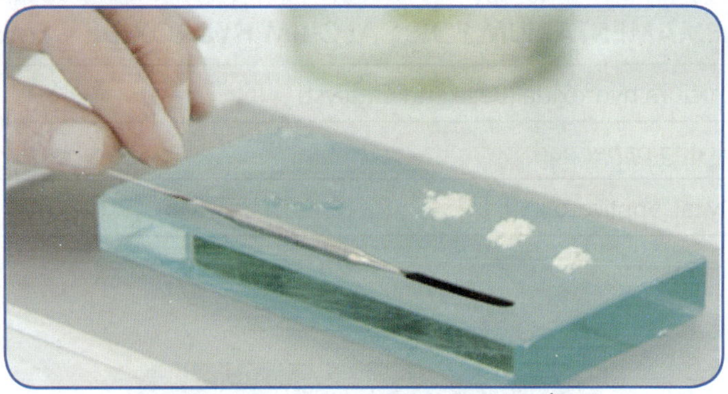

Increments of Powder Before Mixing

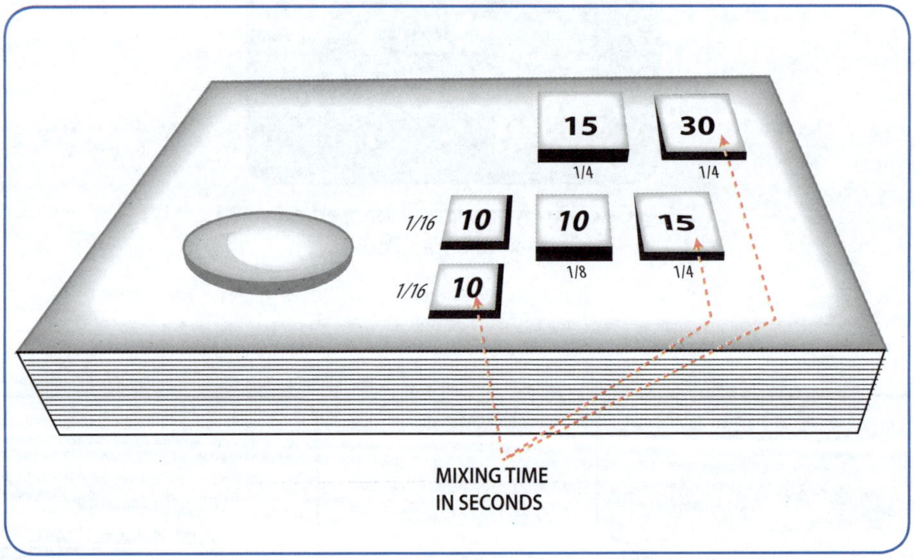

Mixing Time

MIXING

Mixing is done by the slow blending of the segments one at a time. This procedure aids in neutralizing the acid and achieving a smooth consistency. A considerable portion of slab is used. Mixing is done with a moderate circular motion of the spatula blade held flat against the slab. The spatula should be rotated occasionly to blend the material that collects on top of the blade. A good rule is to spatulate the first three segments for about 15 seconds.

The next two segments should be spatulated for about 20 seconds. The final segment should be for 30 to 35 seconds. If this is done, the mixing time is not critical and completion of the mix will take about 1 ½ minutes. It is important to reach the desired consistency by using more powder and not to allow a thinner mix to stiffen by crystallization.

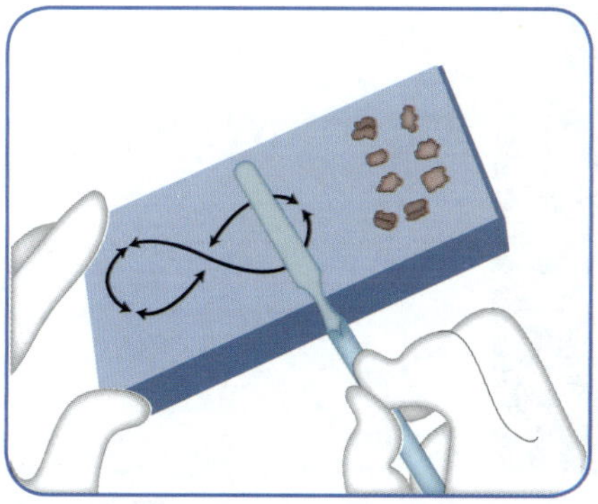

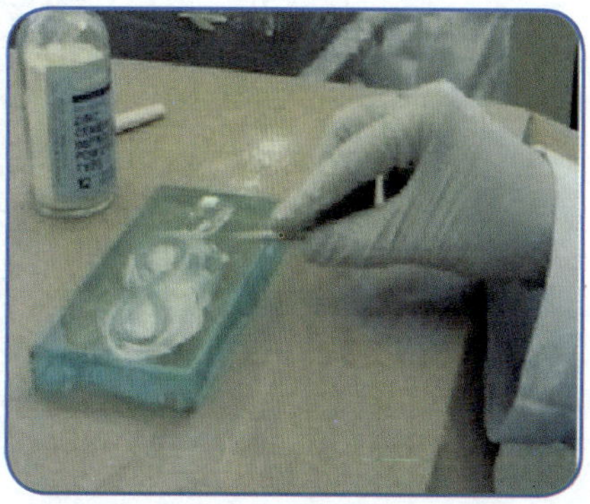

Mixing in Figure 8 Motion

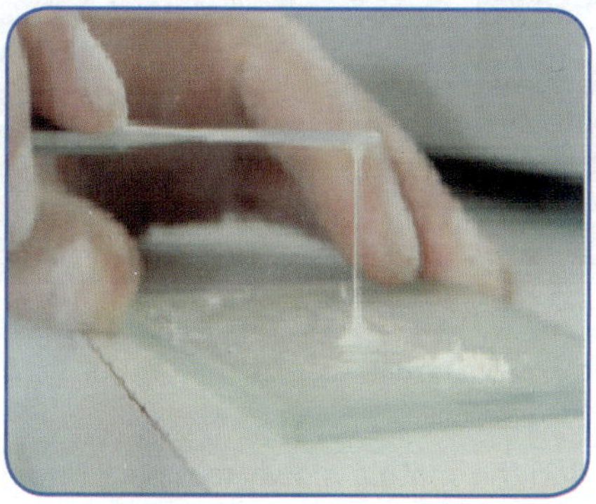

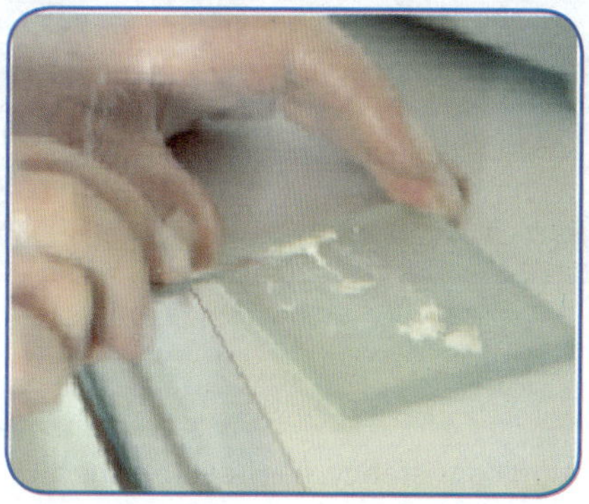

Mixing Showing Thin Consistency

MANIPULATION AND VARIOUS CONSISTENCY OF DENTAL CEMENTS

In order to achieve a homogenous consistency, divide the measured quantity of powder into 4 portions(1/2, 1/4, 1/8, 1/8). Beginning with smallest quantity, blend the powder into the measured liquid within 90 seconds.

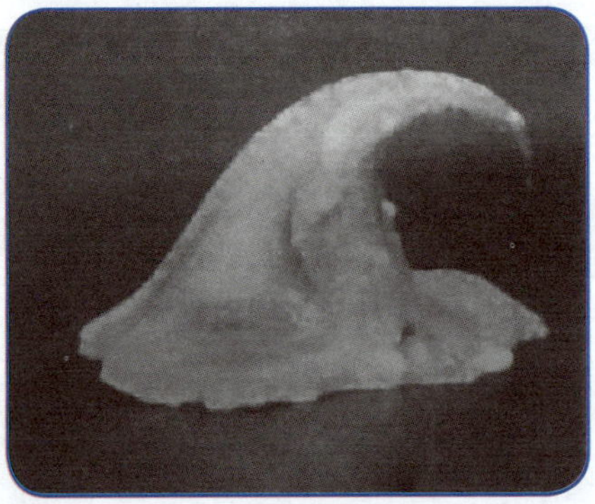

Fig.1

The filling consistency has been reached when on lifting the spatula, the peak drawn out forms a small hook and does not sink back into the paste (Fig 1)

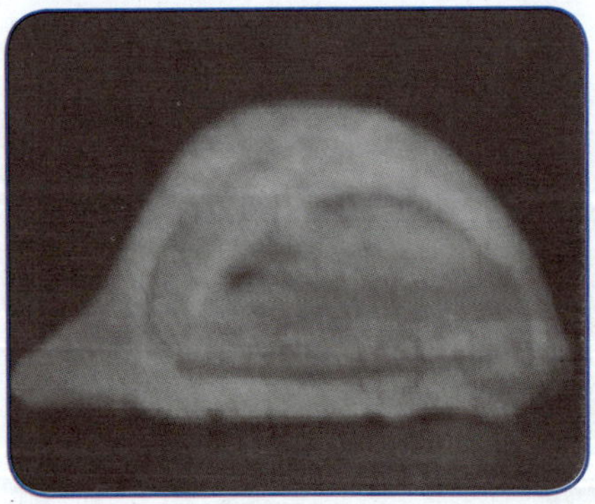

Fig.2

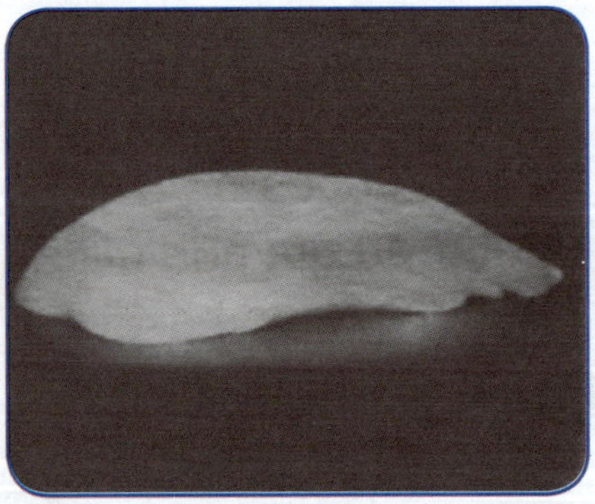

Fig.3

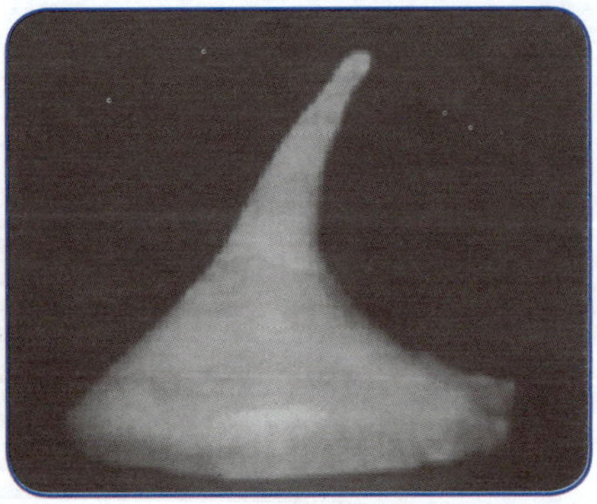

Fig.4

The fixation consistency has been reached when the peak formed on lifting the spatula slowly falls back into the paste (Fig 2, 3 and 4)

PRECAUTIONS FOR MANIPULATION OF DENTAL CEMENTS

Calcium Hydroxide Liner/Base

- Humid conditions will accelerate the setting reaction

Zinc Phosphate Cement

- Do not cool the slab beyond the dew point
- Condensation will adversely affect the mix and setting time
- It is critical to mix the cement slowly, in increments, to dissipate heat
- Make sure the bottles are always properly closed to prevent absorption of moisture

Glass Ionomer Cement

- The mix must be used while it is glossy

Zinc Oxide Eugenol (ZOE) Cement

- For a base consistency, it is important that enough powder is incorporated. Otherwise, the mixture will be sticky and difficult to place

Temporary Cement

- Humidity will accelerate the setting of ZOE based materials

10 PRACTICAL MANIPULATION OF PERMANENT RESTORATIVE MATERIALS

Student Name:____________________________ **Date:**____________________

STEPS OF MANIPULATION FOR DENTAL AMALGAM FILLING

Satisfactory performance of this lab/clinical skill is expected. The student is to self evaluate the designated column. After faculty evaluation, the skill performance is to be discussed based on both evaluations.

If satisfactory, the skill evaluation is complete. If unsatisfactory, remediation will occur until criteria is performed satisfactorily.

CRITERIA	INSTRUCTOR		STUDENT	
	S	U	S	U
1. Proportionating and Dispensing				
2. Trituration				
3. Condensation				
4. Carving				
5. Polishing				

Faculty please identify minimum lab and clinical competency levels:

Laboratory: #____________ criteria must be performed satisfactorily

Clinical: #____________ criteria must be performed satisfactorily

Time Started: ____________ Time Completed: ____________

Instructor Remarks: ________________________

Suggestions/Comments:

____

____

____

____

Student Name:____________________________ **Date:**____________________

AMALGAM FINISHING AND POLISHING

Satisfactory performance of this lab/clinical skill is expected. The student is to self evaluate the designated column. After faculty evaluation, the skill performance is to be discussed based on both evaluations.

If satisfactory, the skill evaluation is complete. If unsatisfactory, remediation will occur until criteria is performed satisfactorily.

CRITERIA	INSTRUCTOR		STUDENT	
	S	U	S	U
Finishing				
1. Excessive amalgam has been removed from the cavosurface margins				
2. Amalgam appears smooth				
3. Occlusion registers properly with articulating paper				
4. Occlusal and marginal anatomy well defined				
5. Porosity and pits have been removed				
6. Contour of the restoration approximates the original contour of the tooth				
7. Adjacent tooth structure have been left undamaged				
Polishing				
1. Amalgam is void of scratches and appears smooth				
2. Amalgam has high polish and lustrous shine				
3. Adjacent tooth structure is left undamaged				
4. Time utilization is satisfactory				

Faculty please identify minimum lab and clinical competency levels:

Laboratory: #______________ criteria must be performed satisfactorily

Clinical: #______________ criteria must be performed satisfactorily

Time Started: ________________ Time Completed: ________________

Instructor Remarks: ____

Suggestions/Comments:

____

____

____

ARMAMENTARIUM FOR DENTAL AMALGAM FILLING
Mercury and dispenser
Matrix band retainer
Silver alloy powder
Articulating paper
Amalgam capsule
Amalgam carrier
Amalgamator
Matrix band
Condenser
Burnisher
Mortar
Carver
Pestle

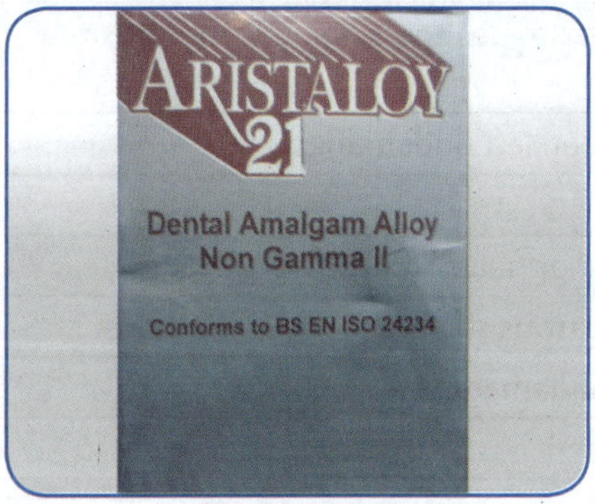

Silver Alloy Powder

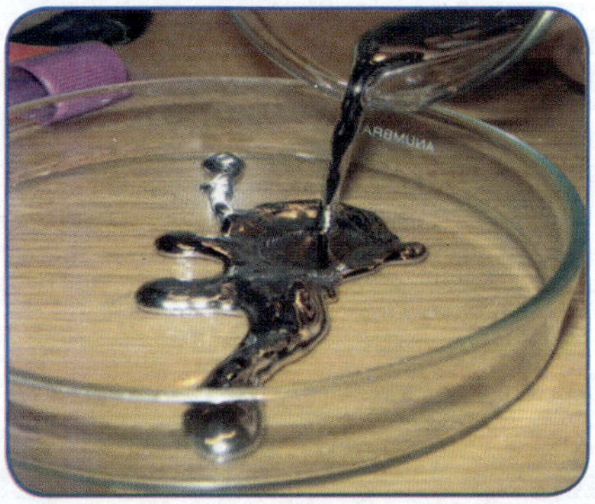

Mercury

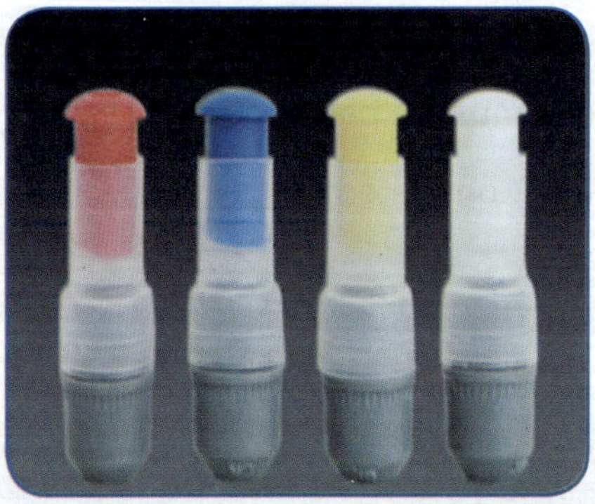

Dental Amalgam Capsules

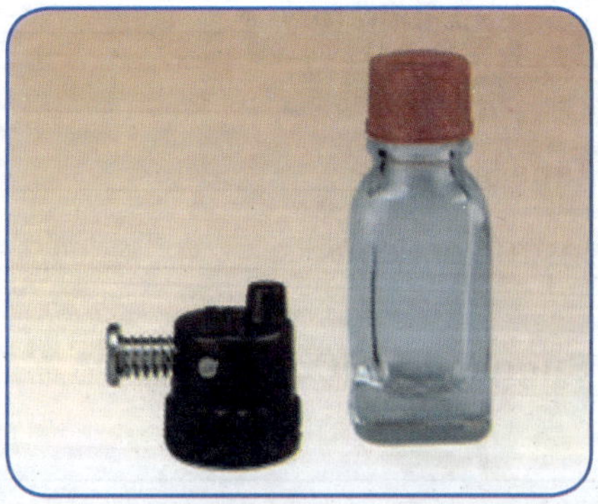

Mercury Dispenser

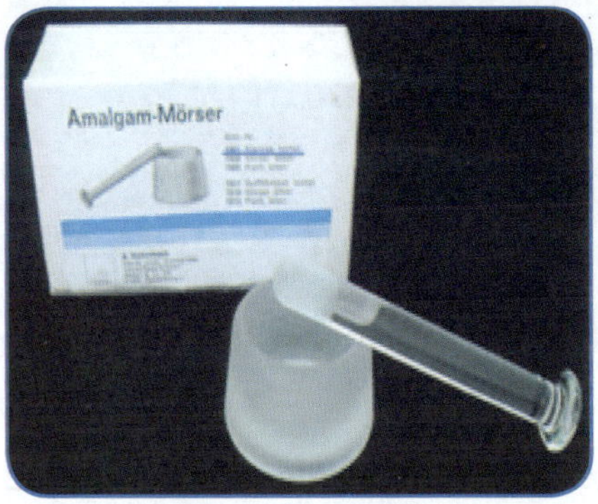

Mortar and Pestle

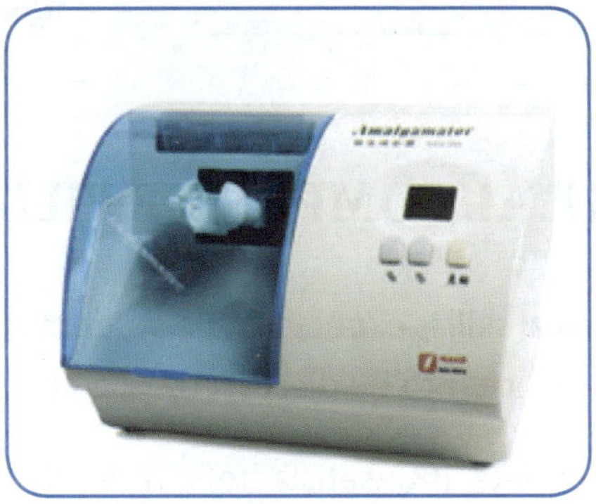

Amalgamator

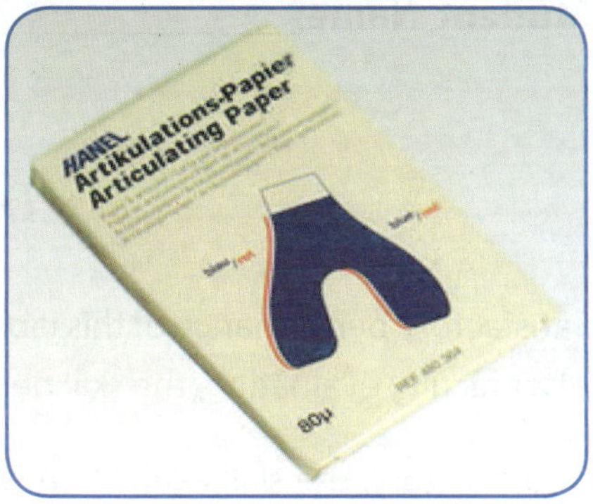

Articulating Paper

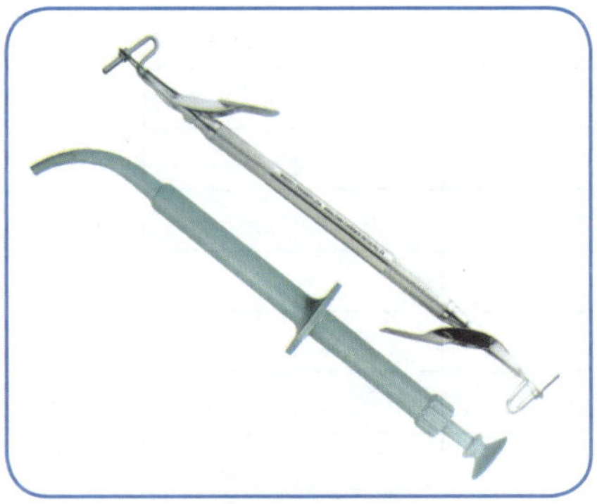

Amalgam Carrier

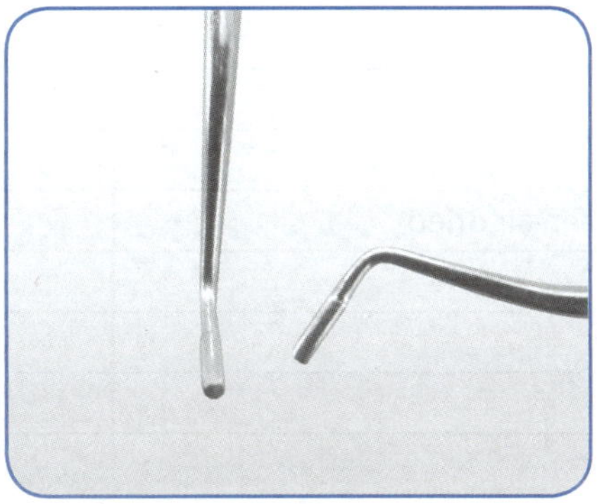

Condenser

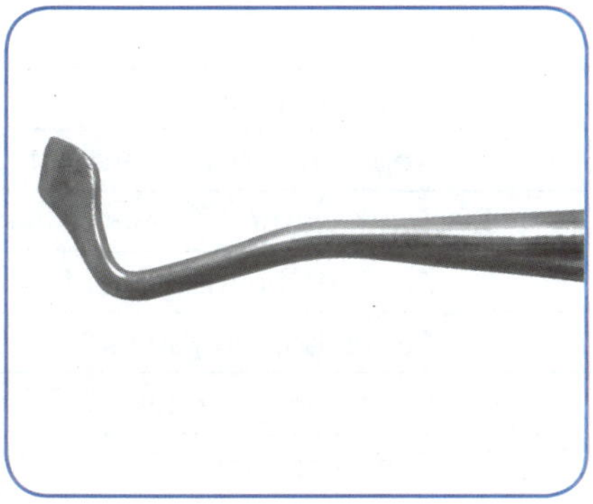

Carver

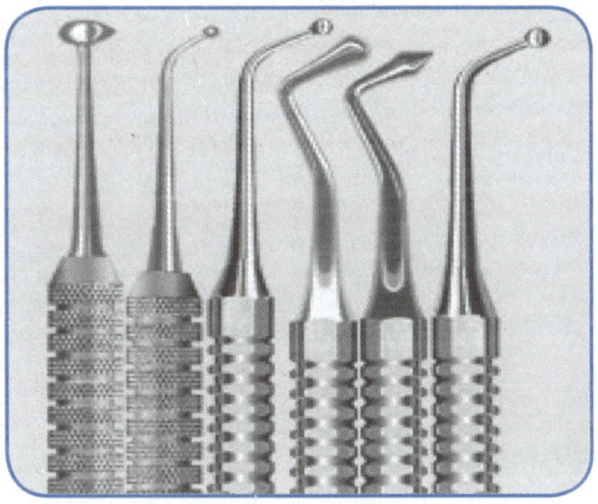

Burnisher

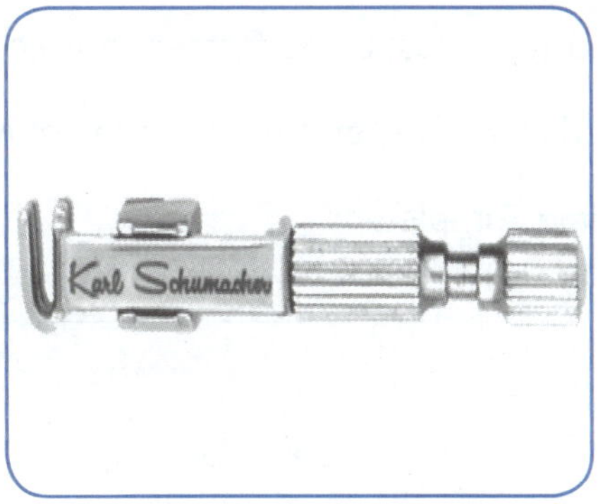

Matrix Band Retainer

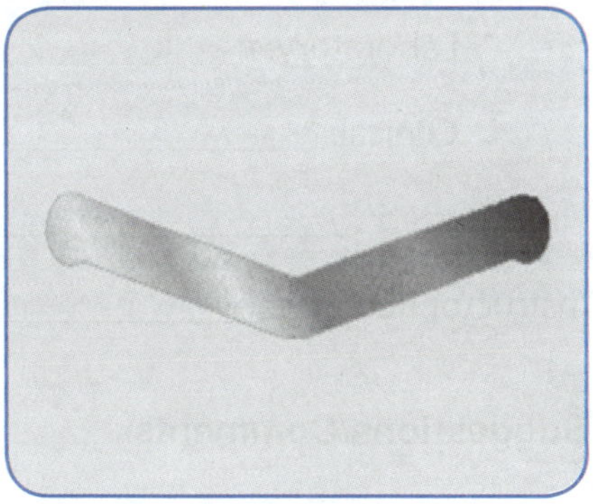

Matrix Band

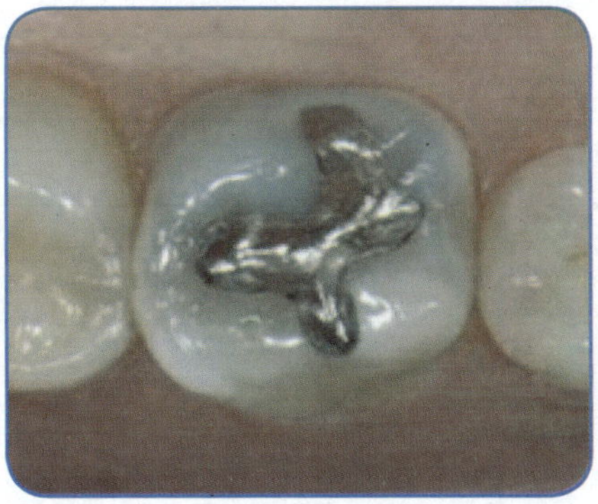

Amalgam Restoration

Student Name:__________________________________ **Date:**_______________________

DENTAL COMPOSITE FILLING

Satisfactory performance of this lab/clinical skill is expected. The student is to self evaluate the designated column. After faculty evaluation, the skill performance is to be discussed based on both evaluations.

If satisfactory, the skill evaluation is complete. If unsatisfactory, remediation will occur until criteria is performed satisfactorily.

CRITERIA	INSTRUCTOR		STUDENT	
	S	U	S	U
1. Preparation of tooth				
2. Application of acid etchant				
3. Tooth washed to remove acid, then air dried				
4. Applying bonding agent				
5. Curing bonding agent				
6. Placement of Composite				
7. Curing of Composite				

Faculty please identify minimum lab and clinical competency levels:

Laboratory: #______________ criteria must be performed satisfactorily

Clinical: #______________ criteria must be performed satisfactorily

Time Started: __________________ Time Completed: ___________________

Instructor Remarks: ____

Suggestions/Comments:

____

____

____

____

ARMAMENTARIUM FOR DENTAL COMPOSITE FILLING
Dental composite tube (Single paste)
Bonding agent/primer
Composite burnisher
Plastic instrument
Protective glasses
Curing light
Acid etchant
Applicator

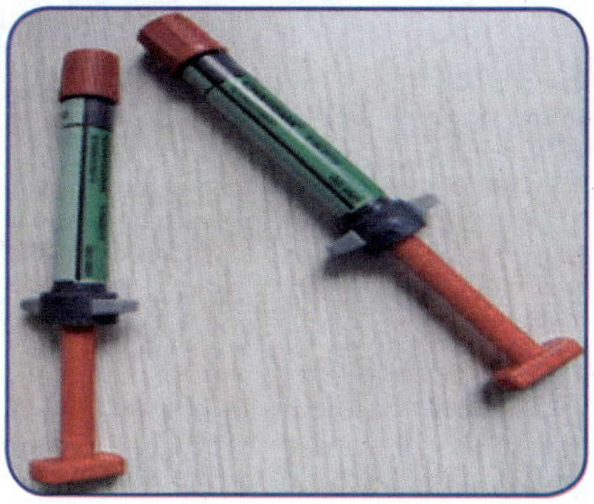

Light Cure Composite

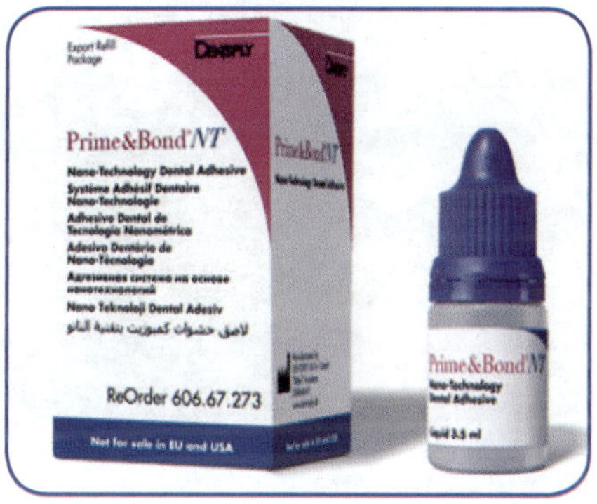

Primer

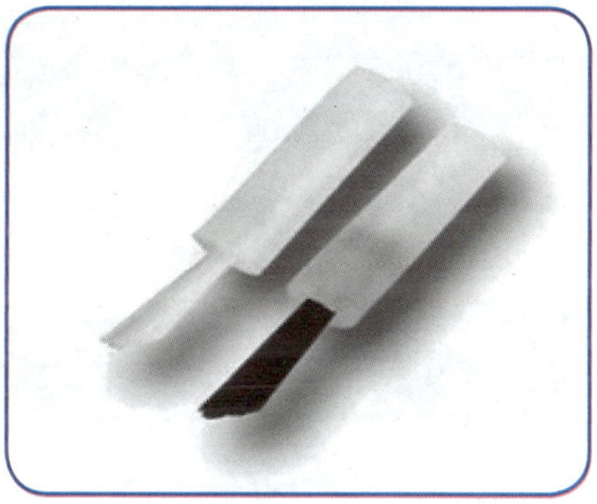

Applicator

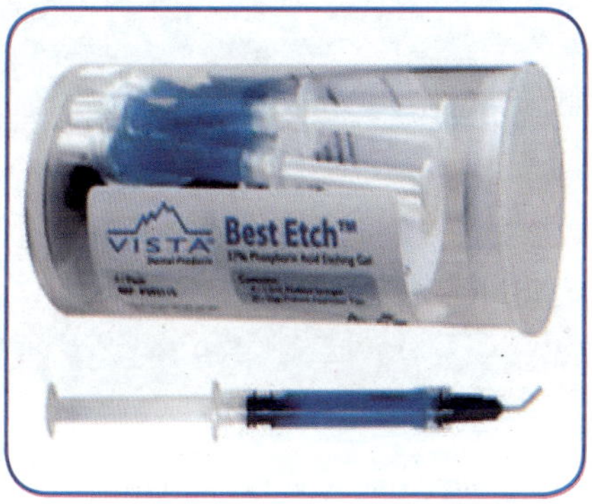

Phosphoric Acid

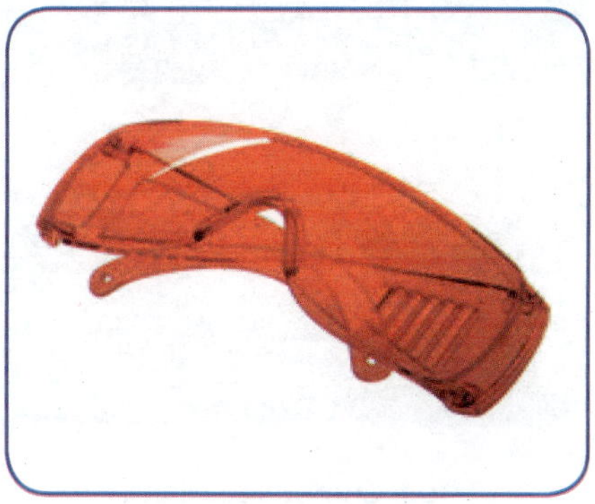

Protective Glasses

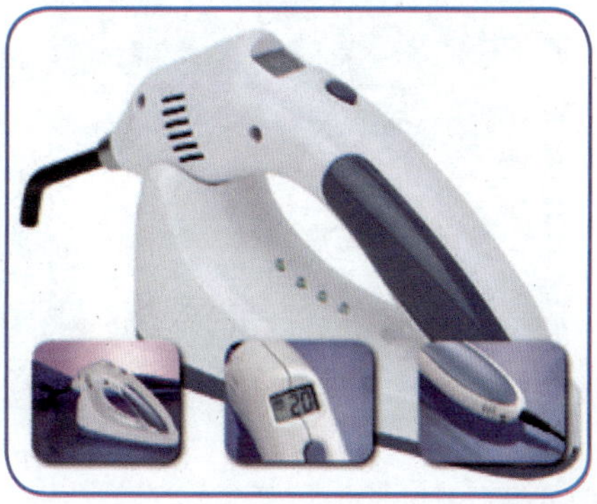

Curing Light

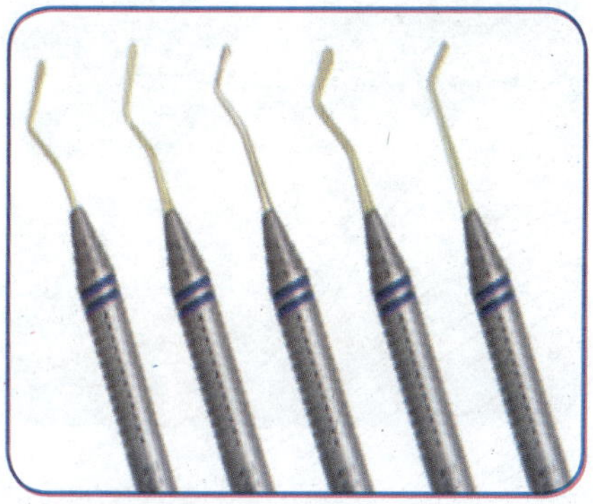

Composite Burnisher

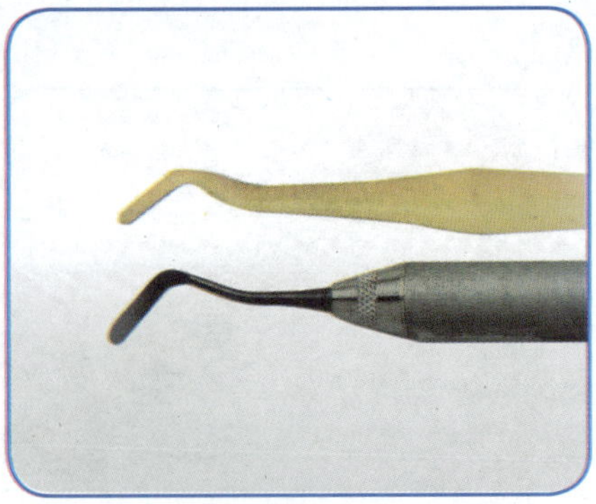

Plastic Instrument

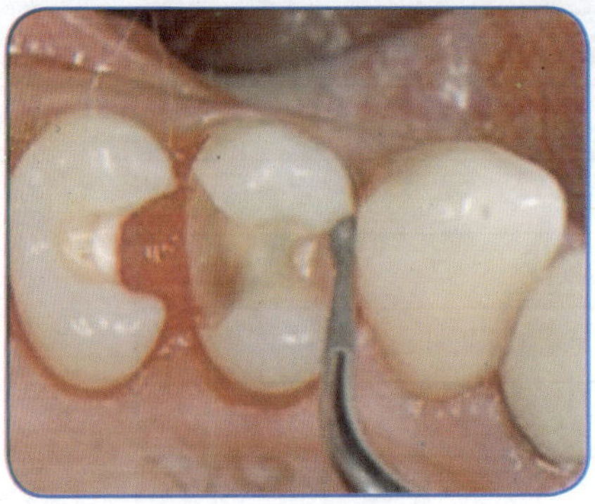

Fig.1 Preparation of Cavity

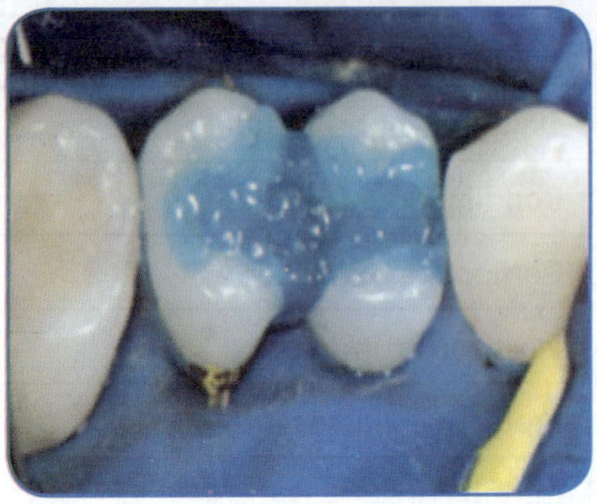

Fig.2 Application of Acid Etchant

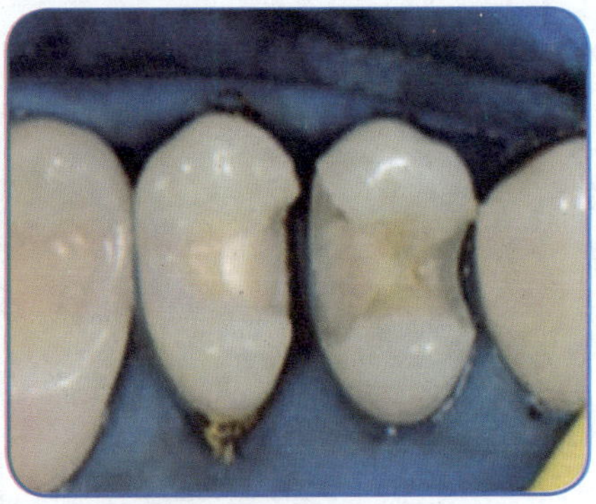

Fig.3 Cavity Wash and Dried

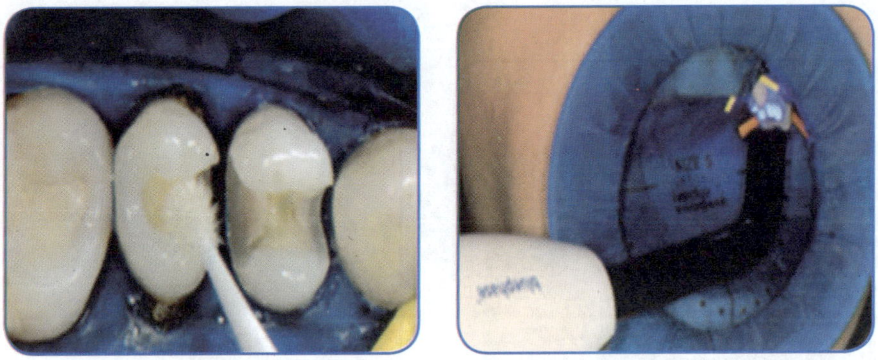

Fig.4 Application of Primer and Light Cure

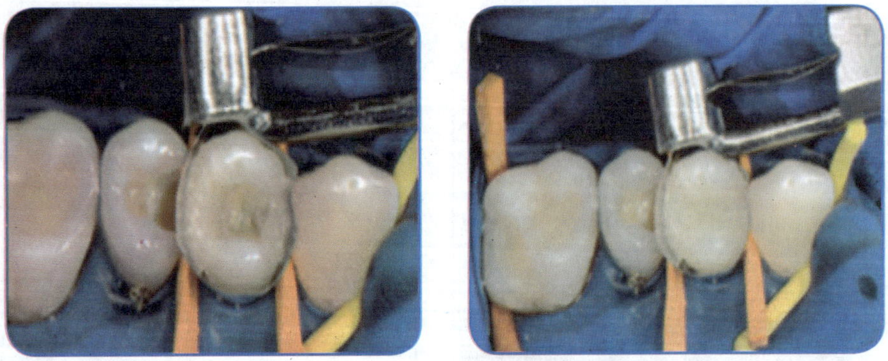

Fig.5 Preparing the Cavity for Filling

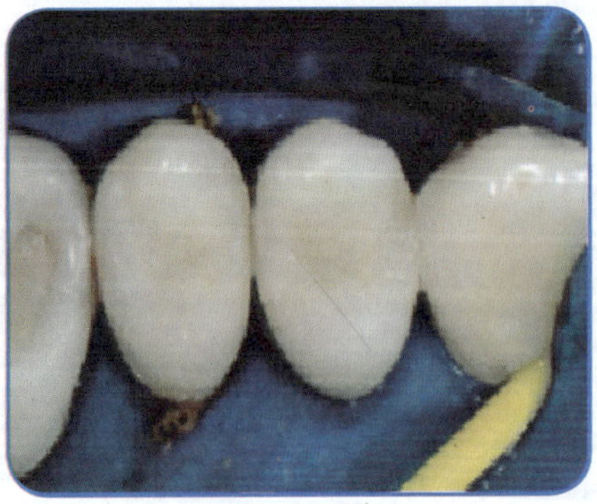

Fig.6 Composite Filling

Student Name:____________________ **Date:**________________

DENTAL COMPOSITE FINISHING AND POLISHING

Satisfactory performance of this lab/clinical skill is expected. The student is to self evaluate the designated column. After faculty evaluation, the skill performance is to be discussed based on both evaluations.

If satisfactory, the skill evaluation is complete. If unsatisfactory, remediation will occur until criteria is performed satisfactorily.

CRITERIA	INSTRUCTOR		STUDENT	
	S	U	S	U
Finishing				
1. Excessive composite have been removed from cavosurface margins				
2. Composite appears to be smooth				
3. Occlusion registers properly with articulating paper				
4. Occlusal and marginal anatomy is well defined				
5. Porosity and pits have been removed				
6. Contour of the restoration approximates the original contour of the tooth				
7. Adjacent tooth structure is left undamaged				
Polishing				
1. Composite is void of scratches and remain smooth				
2. Composite has a lustrous shine				
3. Adjacent tooth structure is left undamaged				
4. Time utilization is satisfactory				

Faculty please identify minimum lab and clinical competency levels:

Laboratory: #____________ criteria must be performed satisfactorily

Clinical: #____________ criteria must be performed satisfactorily

Time Started: ____________ Time Completed: ____________

Instructor Remarks: ________________________

Suggestions/Comments:

ARMAMENTARIUM FOR DENTAL COMPOSITE FINISHING AND POLISHING
Composite finishing kit
Composite polishing kit

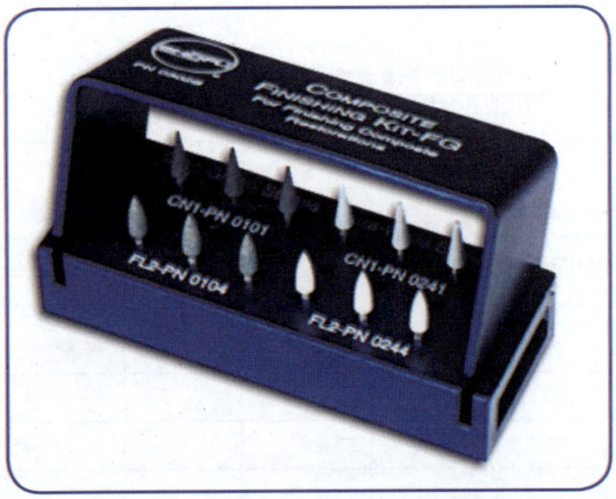

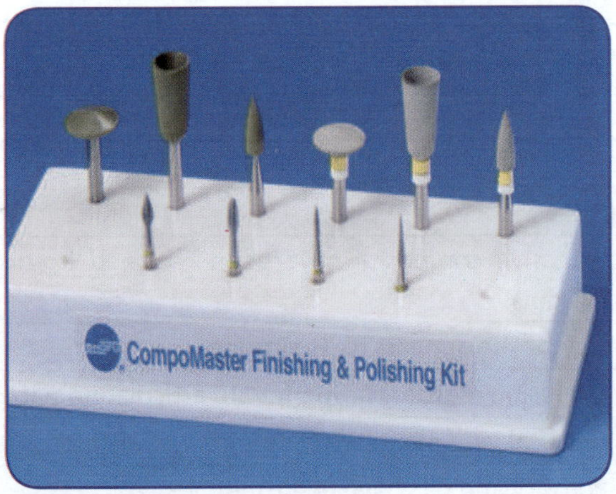

Composite Finishing and Polishing Kit

Section C

11 PRACTICAL

SPECIFICATION FOR MIXING OF ALGINATE POWDER WITH WATER AND ALGINATE IMPRESSION

MIXING RATIO OF ALGINATE POWDER AND WATER

Alginate Powder (gm)		Water (ml)
1	:	2.7 -3
7 gm	:	19 ml

MANUFACTURER'S RECOMMENDED MIXING RATIO

7 gm of Alginate Powder Require 19 ml of Water

WEIGHED AMOUNT OF ALGINATE POWDER OF AVERAGE MAXILLARY ARCH FOR PARTIAL DENTURE IMPRESSION

Alginate Powder =2 scoops =14 gm (1 scoop=7 gm) scoop

Provided by Dental Department

Water = 38 ml

WEIGHED AMOUNT OF ALGINATE POWDER OF AVERAGE MANDIBULAR ARCH FOR PARTIAL DENTURE IMPRESSION

Alginate Powder =1.75 scoops =12.25 gm (1 scoop=7 gm)

Water = 33.25 ml

Student Name:______________________________ **Date:**____________________

ALGINATE IMPRESSION

Satisfactory performance of this lab/clinical skill is expected. The student is to self evaluate the designated column. After faculty evaluation, the skill performance is to be discussed based on both evaluations.

If satisfactory, the skill evaluation is complete. If unsatisfactory, remediation will occur until criteria is performed satisfactorily.

CRITERIA	INSTRUCTOR		STUDENT	
	S	U	S	U
1. All teeth are present without voids and air bubbles				
2. All edentulous ridges are present				
3. All vestibular areas are present and intact				
4. All frenas and muscle attachments are present and intact				
5. All interpapillary spaces are present with minimal tearing				
6. No voids in critical areas: palate, floor of mouth, vestibular areas, tray showing through impression				
7. Impression is stable, alginate is attached to the tray				
8. Adequately extended retromolar area included				
9. Appropriate infection control procedures: bowls, spatula and impressions				

Faculty please identify minimum lab and clinical competency levels:

Laboratory: #____________ criteria must be performed satisfactorily

Clinical: #____________ criteria must be performed satisfactorily

Time Started: ________________ Time Completed: ________________

Instructor Remarks: ______________________________________

Suggestions/Comments:

____

____

____

____

ARMAMENTARIUM FOR DENTAL ALGINATE IMPRESSION
Maxillary and Mandibular impression trays
Room temperature water
Water measuring cylinder
Alginate Mixing bowl
Wide blade spatula
Weighing balance
Alginate powder

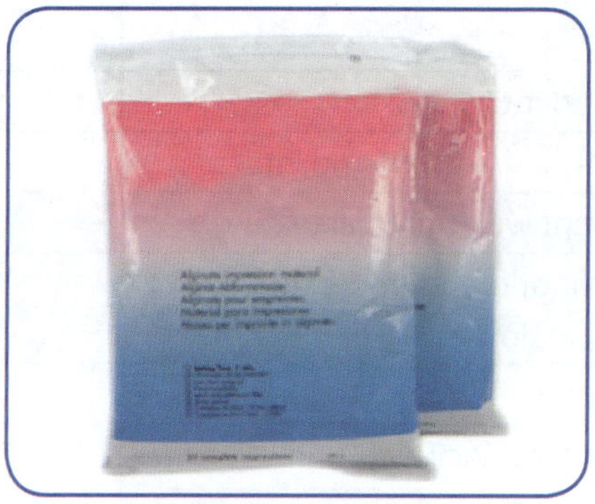

Alginate Powder

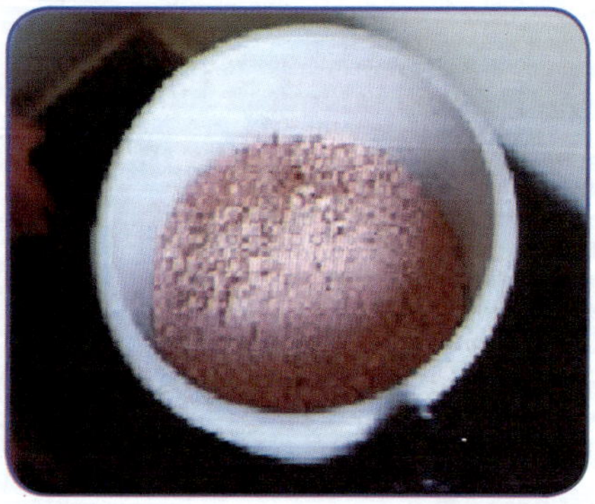

Alginate Powder in Rubber Bowl

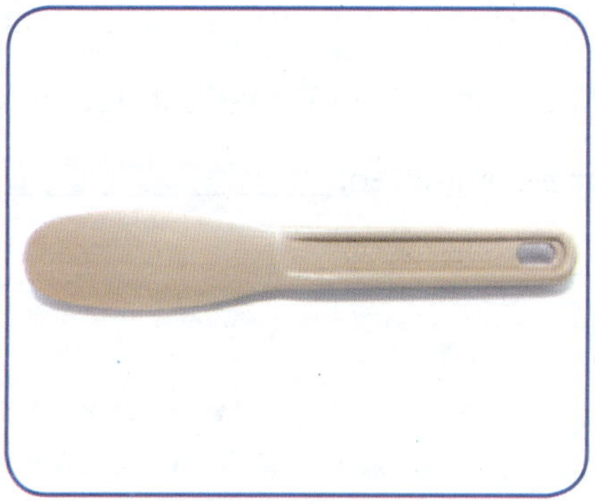

Wide Blade Spatula

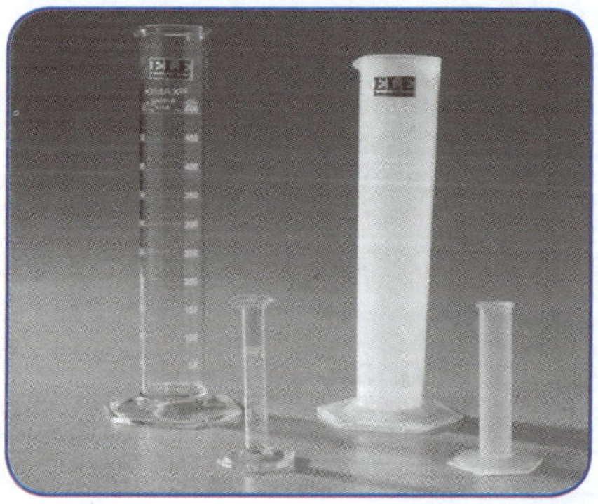

Water Measuring Cylinder

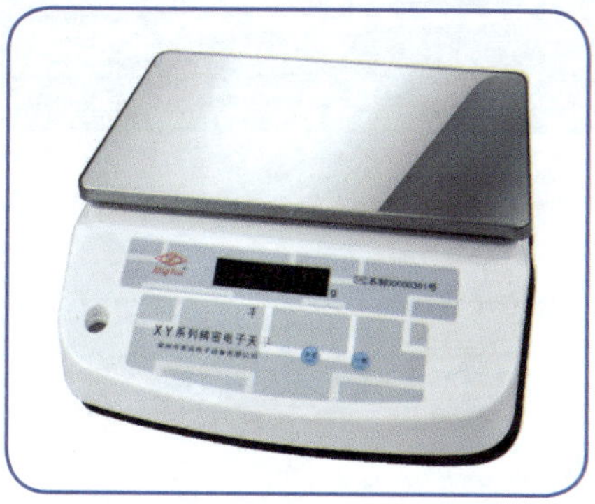

Weighing Balance

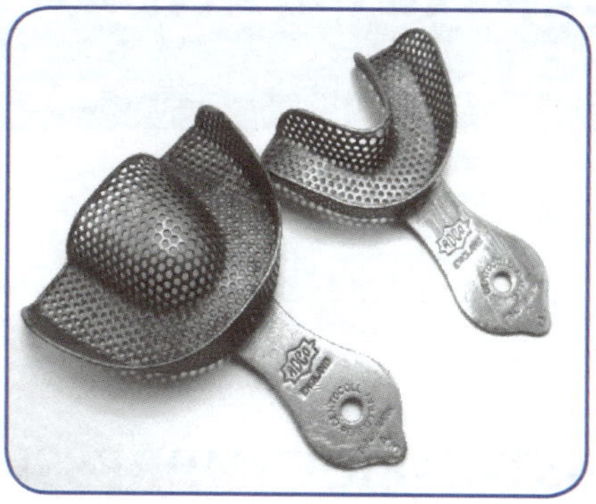

Impression Tray

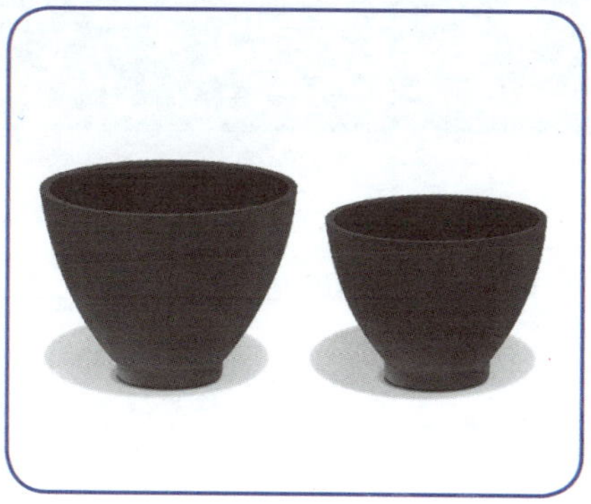

Rubber Bowl

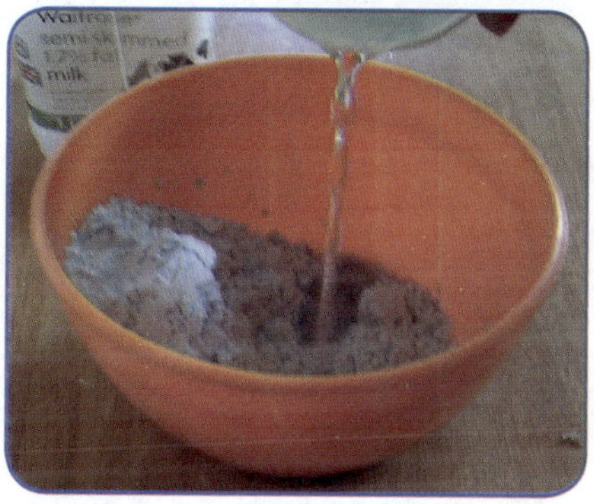

Pouring Water

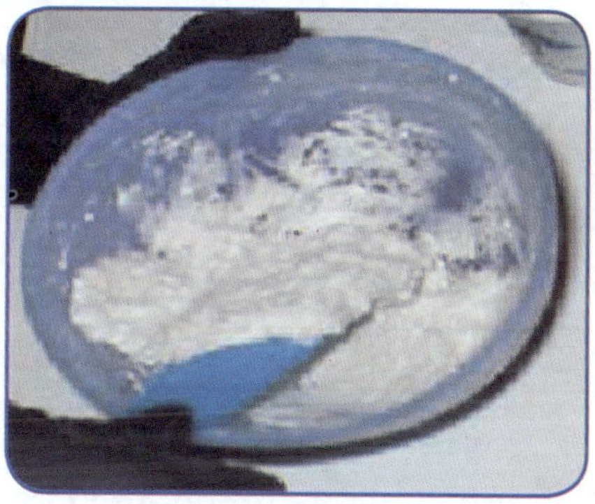

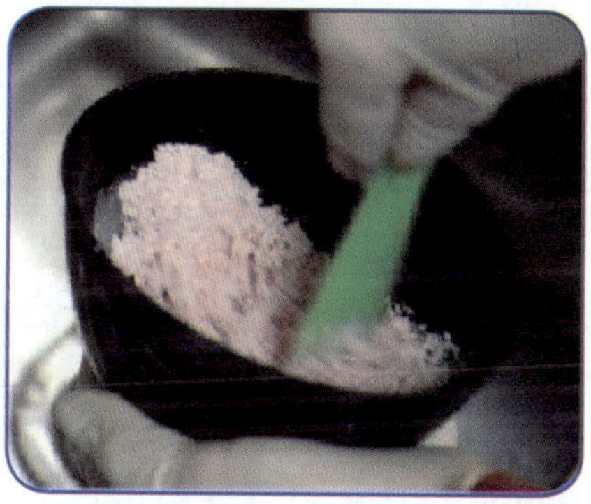

Mixing Alginate Powder

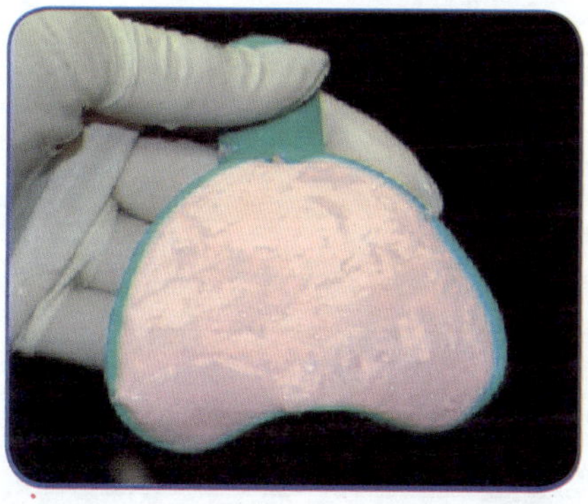

Loading Impression Material on to Tray

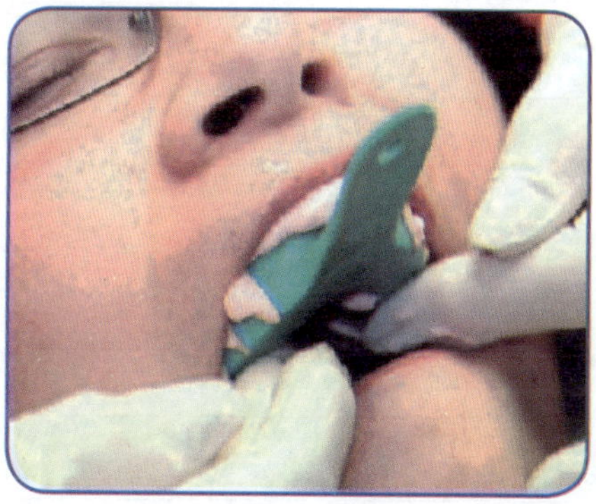

Tray Placed in Oral Cavity

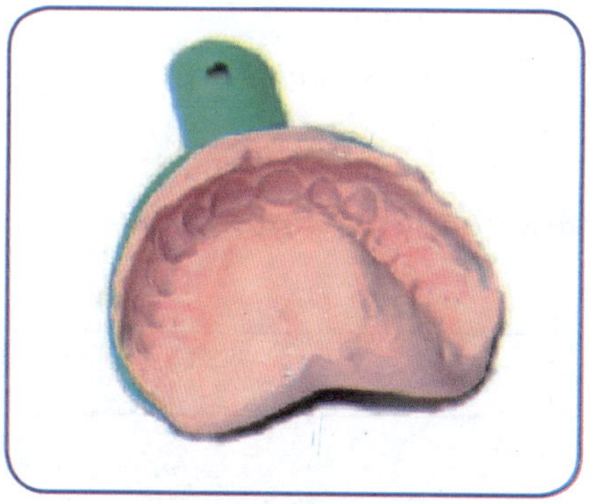

Maxillary Impression

12 PRACTICAL ELASTOMERIC IMPRESSIONS

Student Name:________________________________ **Date:**________________________

ELASTOMERIC IMPRESSIONS

Satisfactory performance of this lab/clinical skill is expected. The student is to self evaluate the designated column. After faculty evaluation, the skill performance is to be discussed based on both evaluations.

If satisfactory, the skill evaluation is complete. If unsatisfactory, remediation will occur until criteria is performed satisfactorily.

CRITERIA	INSTRUCTOR		STUDENT	
	S	U	S	U
1. No bubbles or voids are present in critical areas				
2. Impression is not distorted				
3. All critical areas are reproduced				
4. No critical areas are torn				

Faculty please identify minimum lab and clinical competency levels:

Laboratory: #_______________ criteria must be performed satisfactorily

Clinical: #_______________ criteria must be performed satisfactorily

Time Started: ___________________ Time Completed: _____________________

Instructor Remarks: ____

Suggestions/Comments:

____

____

____

____

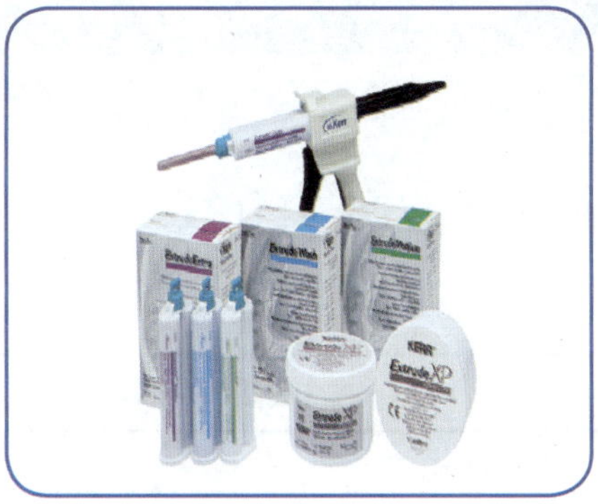

Silicone Heavy, Medium, Light Bodied Impression

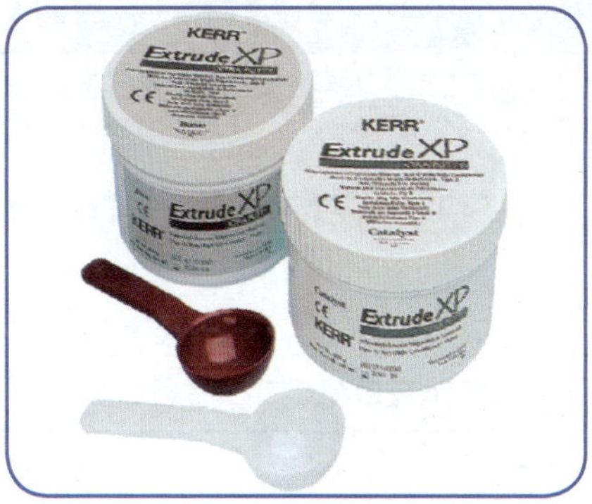

Silicone Putty

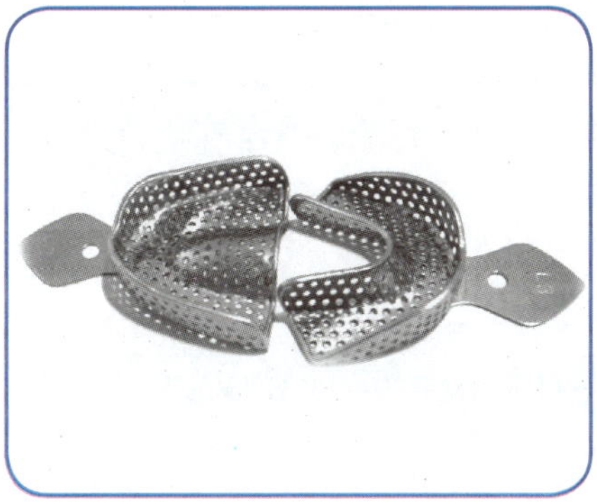

Impression Trays

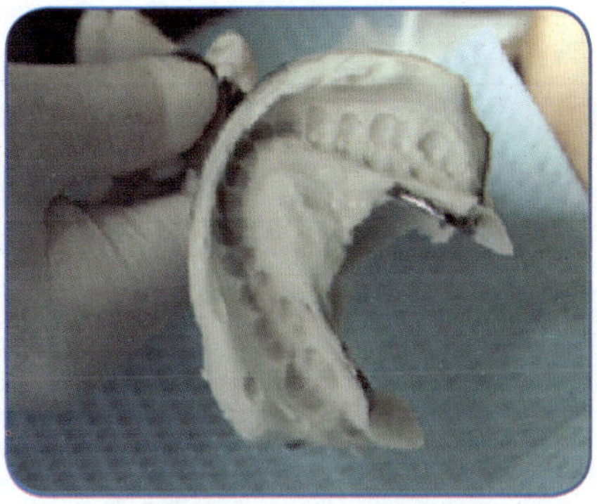

Mandibular Impression

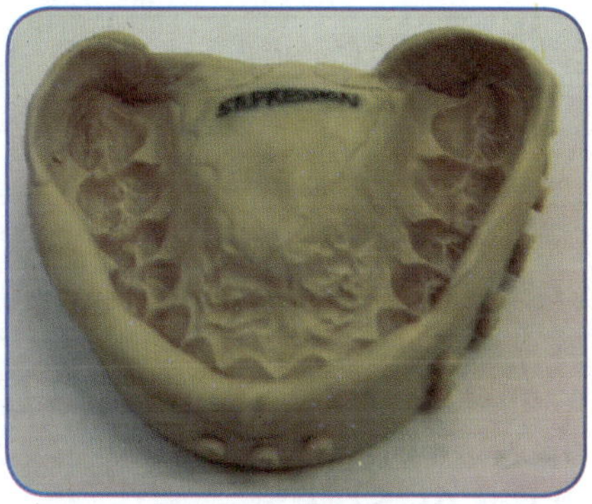

Maxillary Impression

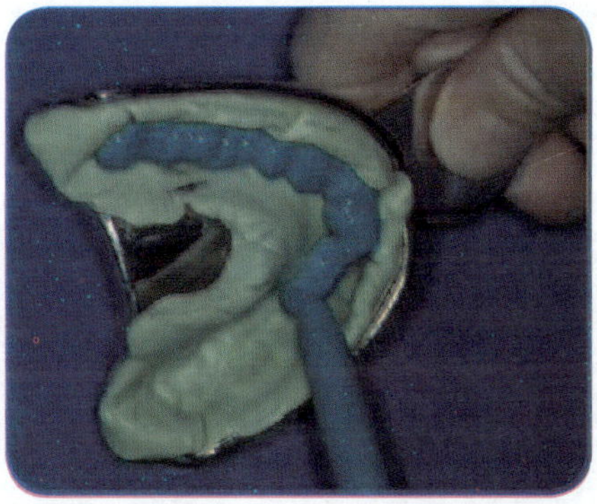

Light Body on Putty Elastomer

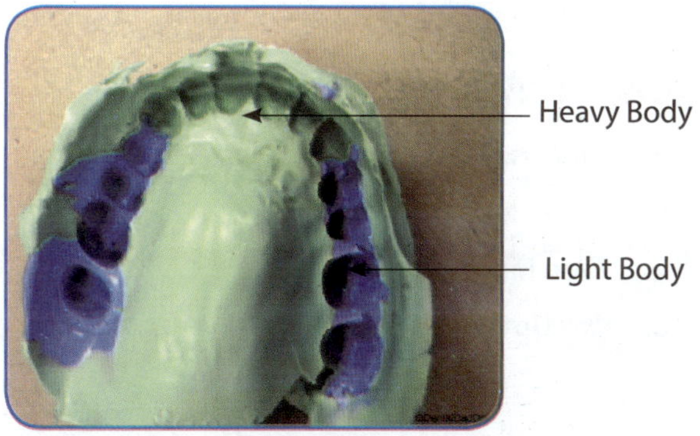

Silicone Impression

13 PRACTICAL

FABRICATION OF ACRYLIC PARTIAL AND COMPLETE DENTURE

REQUIREMENTS FOR MAKING ACRYLIC DENTURE

MATERIALS		EQUIPMENT	
1	Impression Material	1	Curing Flask
2	Soft Plaster/Hard Plaster	2	Bench Press
3	Acrylic Resin(Heat Cured/Auto Cured)	3	Water Bath
4	Modelling Wax	4	Buffing Machine
5	Acrylic Teeth Strip	5	Vibrating Machine
6	Stone and Vulcanite Burs	6	Plaster Trimmer
7	Polishing Material		

DEMONSTRATION

STEPS FOR MAKING OF ACRYLIC PARTIAL DENTURE

CLINICAL STEPS

1. Patient's History
2. Examination (Intra Oral and Extra Oral)
3. Selection of Trays
4. Taking Impression (Alginate Impression Material)

LABORATORY STEPS

5. Impression Pouring (Hard Plaster/Soft Plaster)
6. Plaster Model
7. Clasp Making if Required
8. Wax Up

CLINICAL STEP

9. Bite Registration

LABORATORY STEP

10. Articulation

CLINICAL STEP

11. Trial

LABORATORY STEPS

12. Flasking
13. Dewaxing
14. Packing
15. Curing
16. Polishing and Finishing

CLINICAL STEP

17. Insertion of Acrylic Partial Denture in the Patient's Mouth

STEPS FOR MAKING OF ACRYLIC COMPLETE DENTURE

CLINICAL STEPS

1. Patient's History
2. Examination (Intra Oral and Extra Oral)
3. Selection of Trays
4. Taking Initial Impression (Impression Compound Cake Form)

LABORATORY STEPS

5. Impression Pouring (Soft Plaster)
6. Plaster Model
7. Fabrication of Custom Made Tray (Acrylic)

CLINICAL STEPS

8. Border Trimming (Green Stick Impression Compound) on Custom Made Tray
9. Wash Impression (Zinc Oxide Eugenol Impression Paste) on Custom Made Tray

LABORATORY STEPS

10. Pouring of Impression (Hard Plaster)
11. Fabrication of Acrylic Base Plate
12. Occlusal Rims

CLINICAL STEP

13. Jaw Registration

LABORATORY STEPS

14. Articulation
15. Teeth Set Up

CLINICAL TRAIL

16. Trial

LABORATORY STEPS

17. Flasking
18. Dewaxing
19. Packing (Heat Cure Acrylic)
20. Curing
21. Polishing and Finishing

CLINICAL STEP

22. Insertion of Acrylic Complete Denture in the Patient's Mouth

Student Name:______________________________ **Date:**____________________

FABRICATION OF CUSTOM MADE TRAY

Satisfactory performance of this lab/clinical skill is expected. The student is to self evaluate the designated column. After faculty evaluation, the skill performance is to be discussed based on both evaluations.

If satisfactory, the skill evaluation is complete. If unsatisfactory, remediation will occur until criteria is performed satisfactorily.

CRITERIA	INSTRUCTOR		STUDENT	
	S	U	S	U
1. Tray has uniform thickness				
2. Tray is smooth				
3. Placements of stops are appropriate				
4. Sizes of stops are adequate				
5. Handle size is acceptable				
6. Handle location is acceptable				

Faculty please identify minimum lab and clinical competency levels:

Laboratory: #____________ criteria must be performed satisfactorily

Clinical: #____________ criteria must be performed satisfactorily

Time Started: ______________ Time Completed: ______________

Instructor Remarks: ______________________________

Suggestions/Comments:

____

____

____

____

ARMAMENTARIUM FOR CUSTOM IMPRESSION TRAY
Self Cure Acrylic Powder
Monomer Liquid
Mixing Spatula
Resin Cup

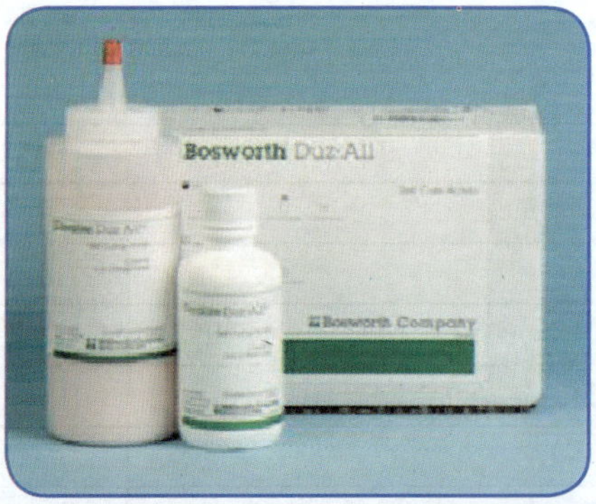

Acrylic Powder and Monomer Liquid

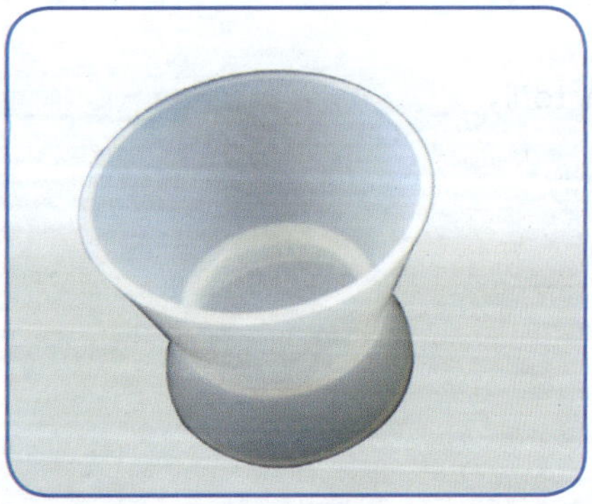

Resin Cup

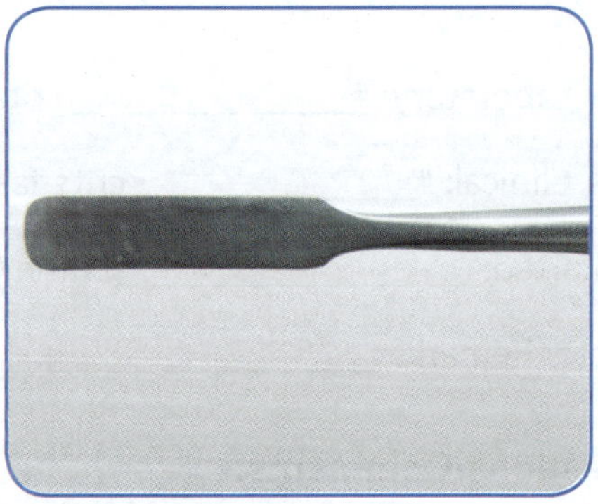

Mixing Spatula

STEPS OF MAKING PARTIAL DENTURE

TRAY SELECTION

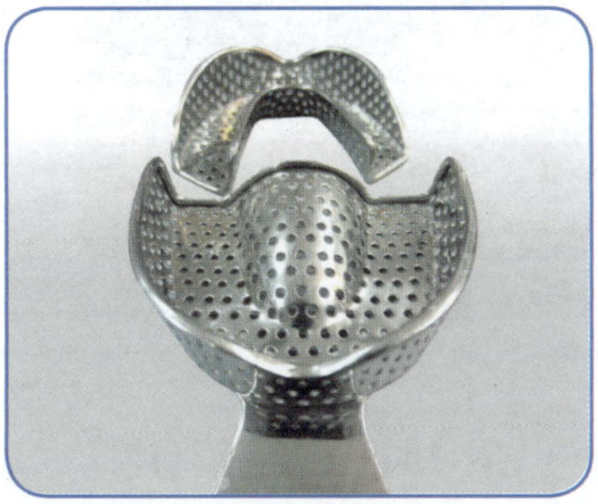

Impression Trays

PREPARATION

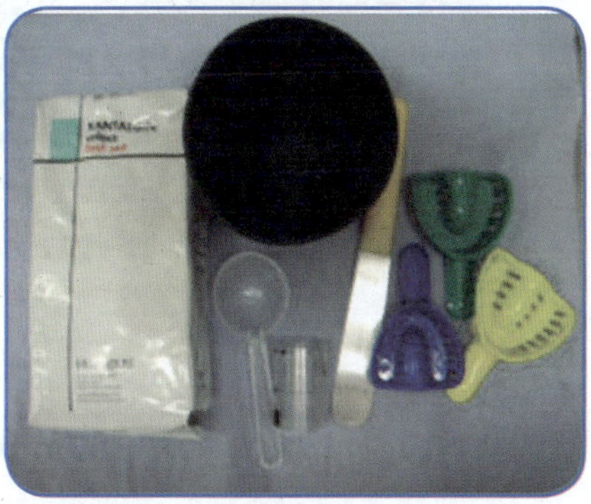

Alginate Powder and Armamentarium Used for Partial Denture Impression

FIRST CLINICAL STEP

IMPRESSION MAKING

MIXING OF ALGINATE

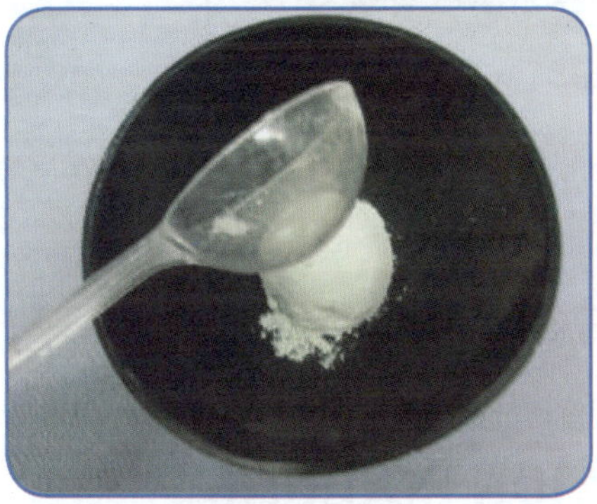

A

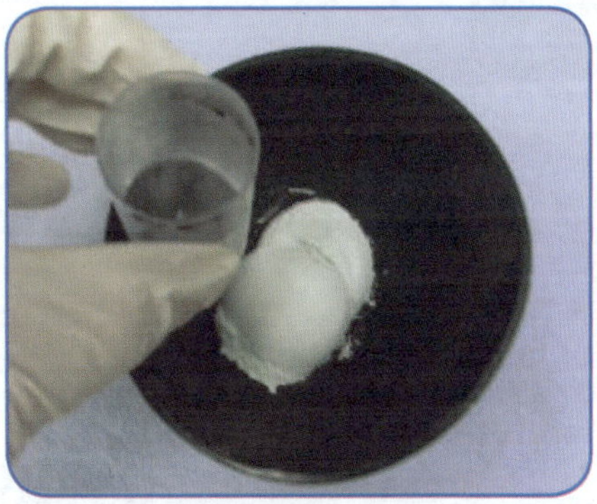

B

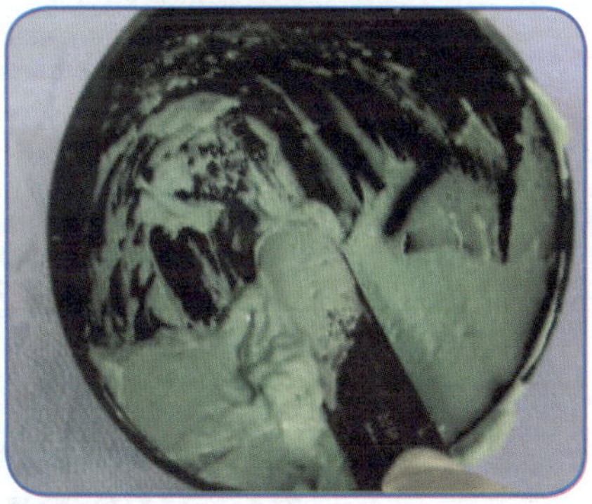

C

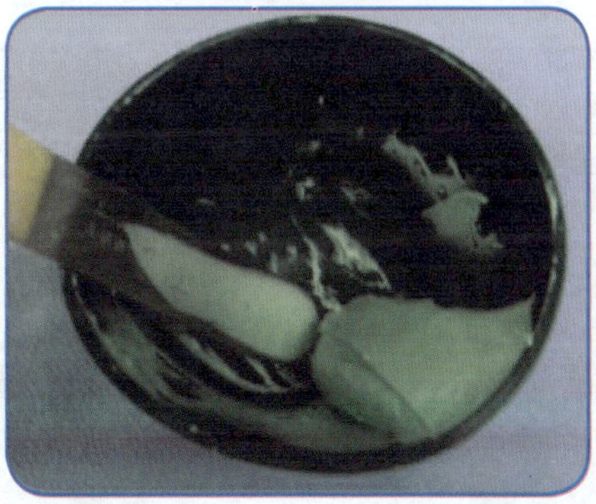

D

LOADING IMPRESSION ON TRAY

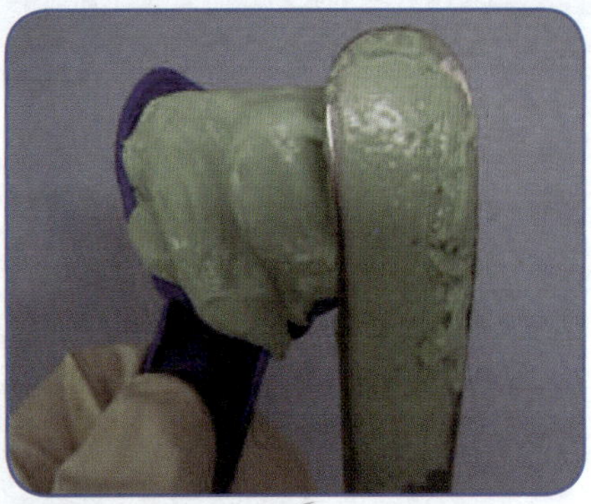

IMPRESSION MAKING

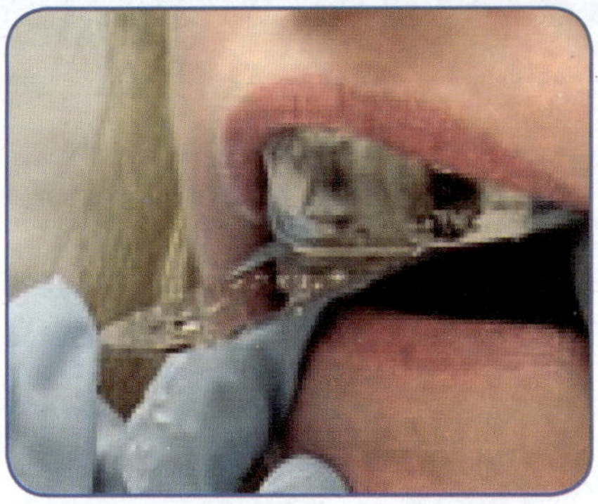

REMOVAL OF TRAY

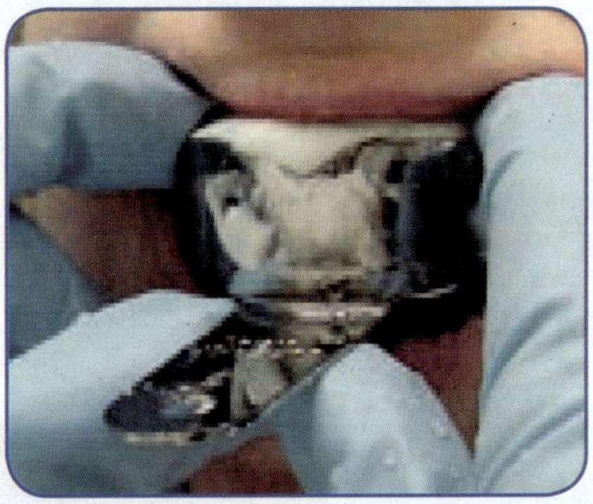

AFTER IMPRESSION

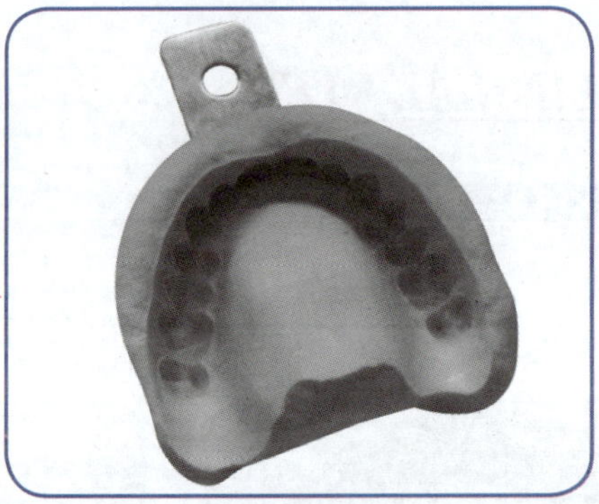

FIRST LABORATORY STEP

AFTER WASHING AND DISINFECTION

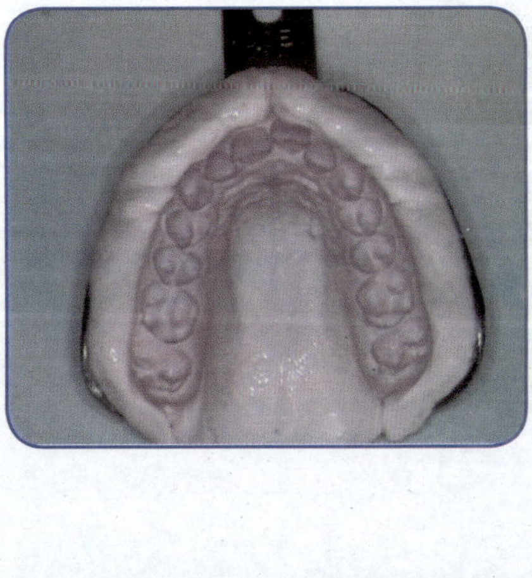

IMPRESSION POURING

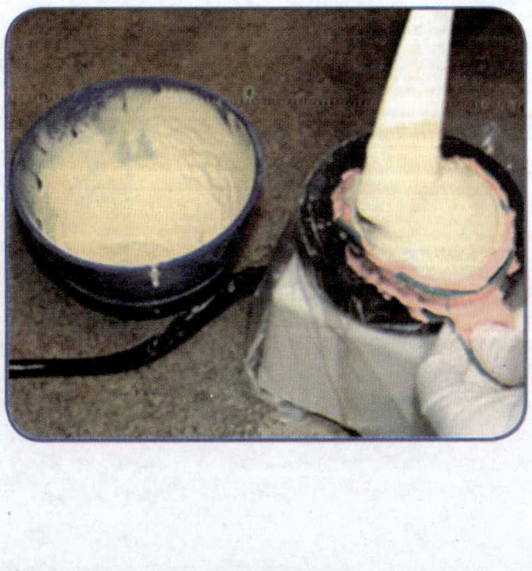

BASE FORMATION

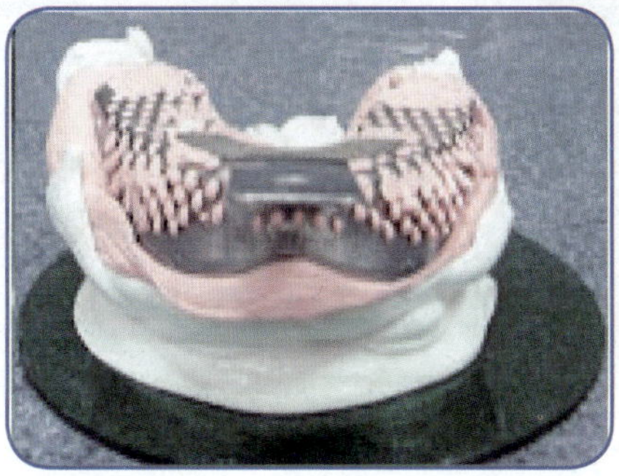

SETTING AND REMOVAL OF THE CAST

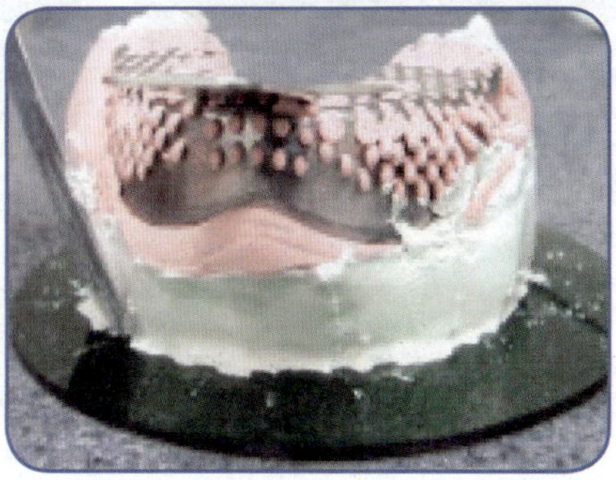

GYPSUM MODEL

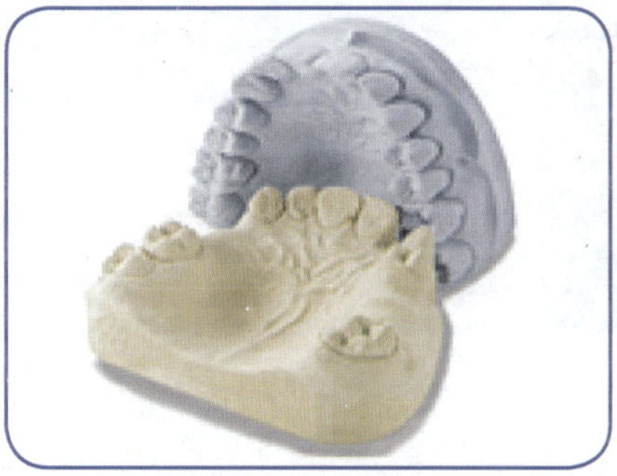

BLOCKOUT THE UNDERCUTS WITH WAX

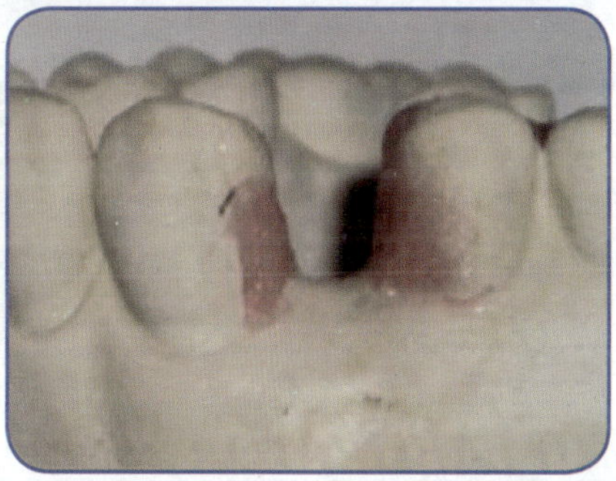

DUPLICATION AFTER BLOCK OUT THE UNDERCUTS

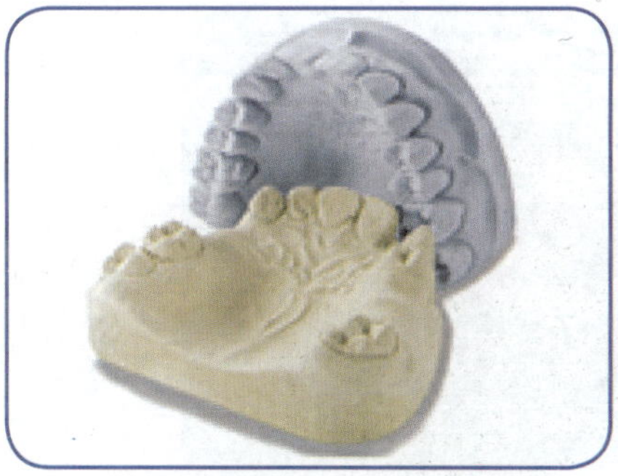

C-CLASP MAKING

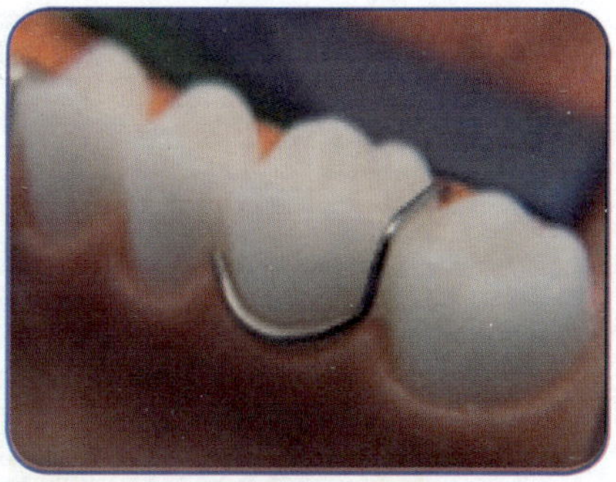

WAX UP AND TEETH ARRANGEMENT

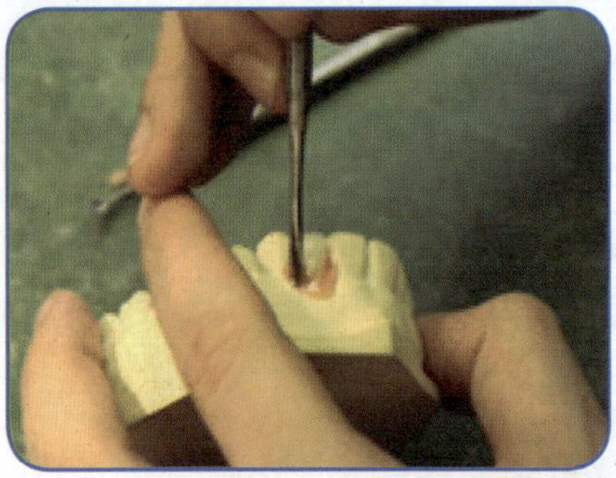
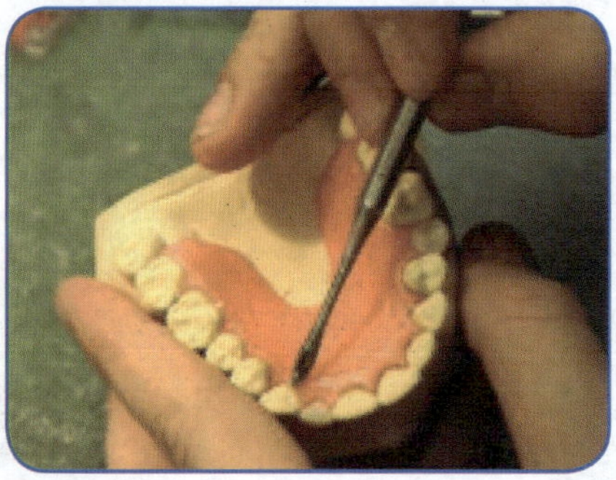
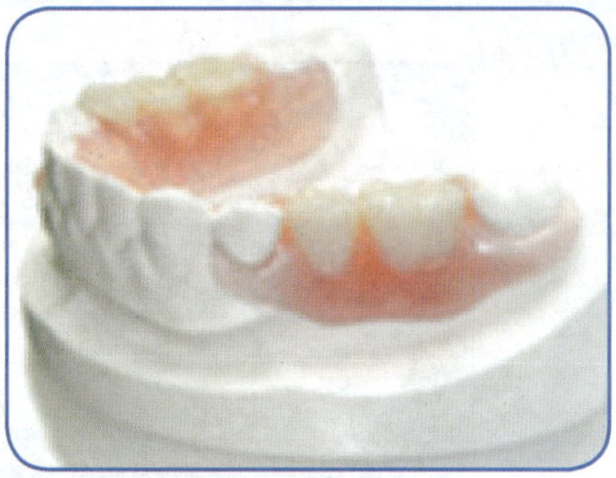

SECOND CLINICAL STEP

DENTURE TRIAL

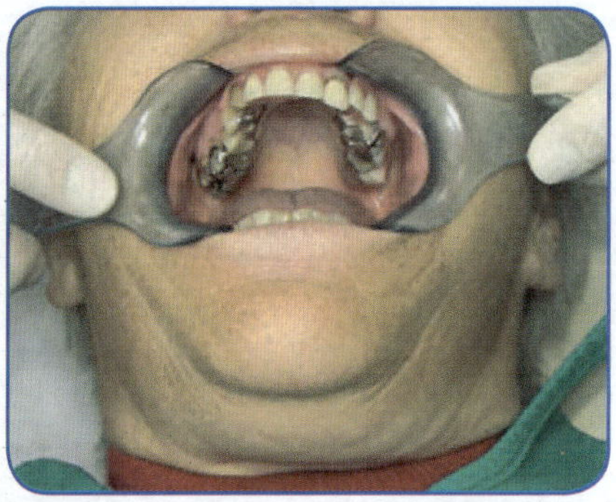

SECOND LABORATORY STEP

DENTURE PROCESSING

FLASKING

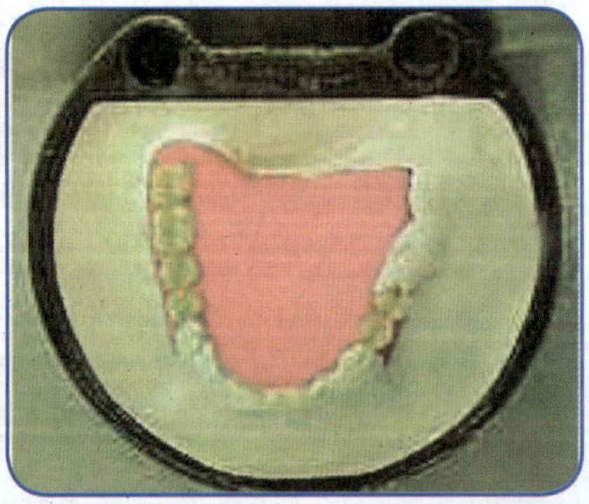

A

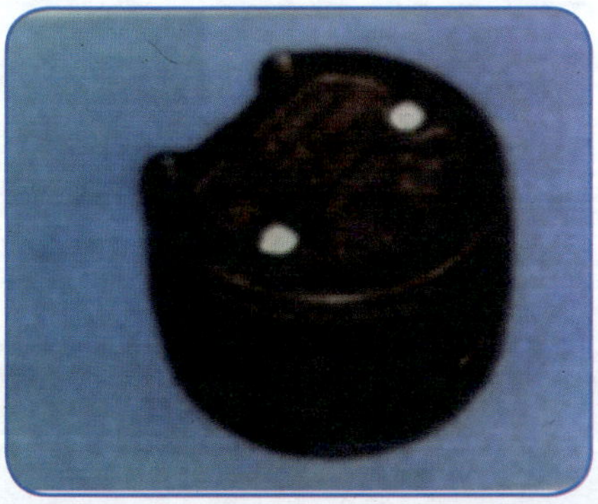

B

DEWAXING

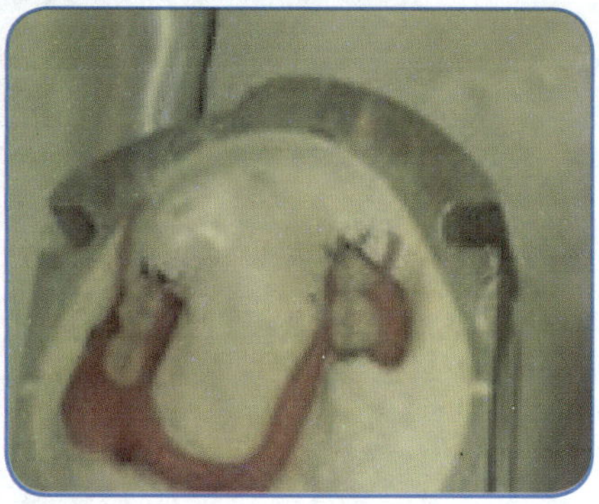

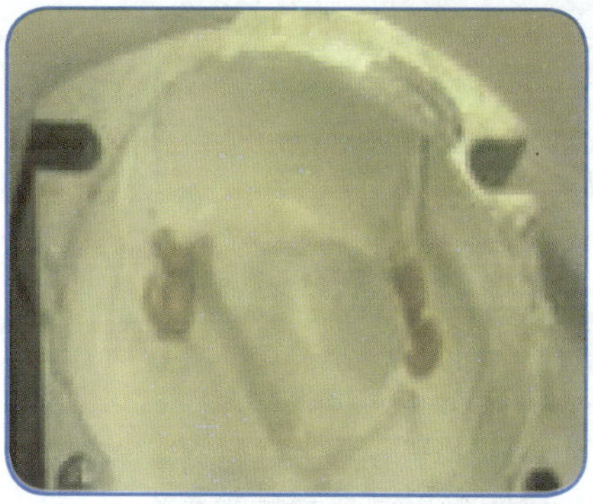

APPLICATION OF COLD MOULD SEAL

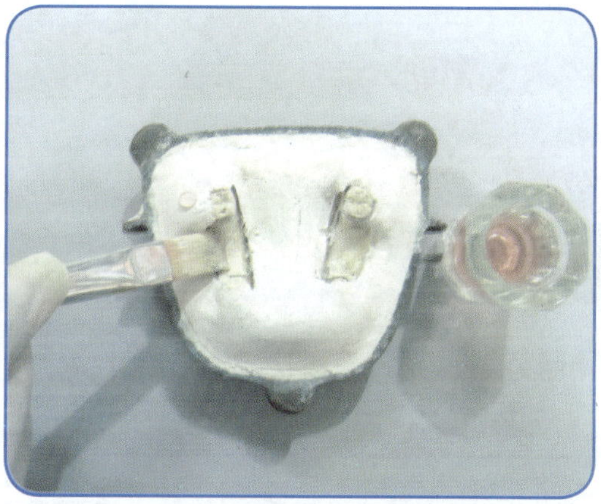

PACKING AND CURING OF ACRYLIC RESIN

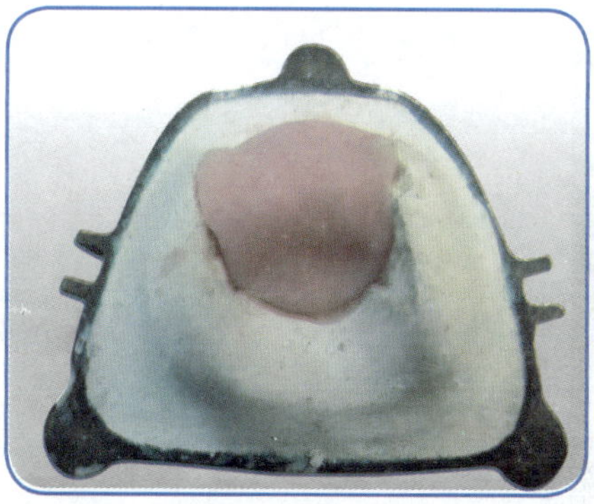

Packing

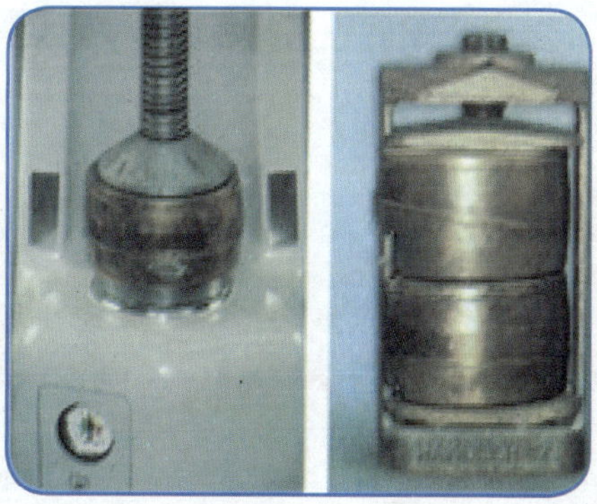

Pressing

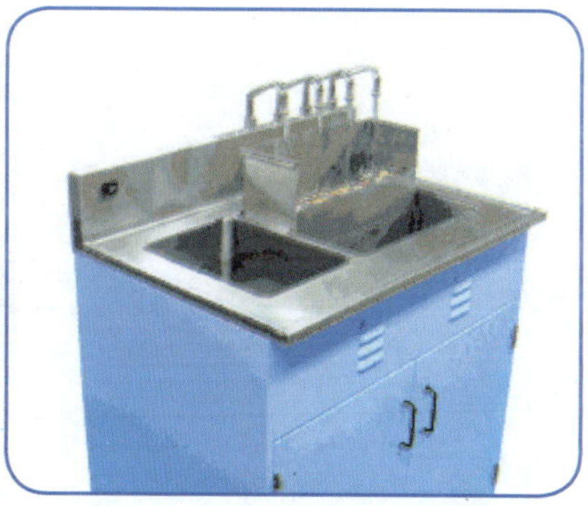

Curing Bath

DENTURE FINISHING AND POLISHING

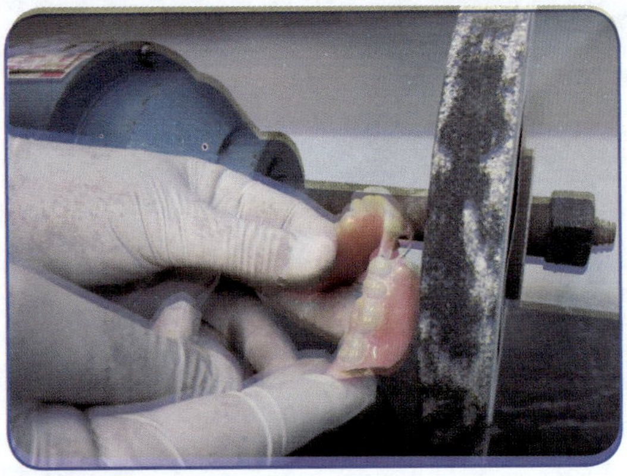

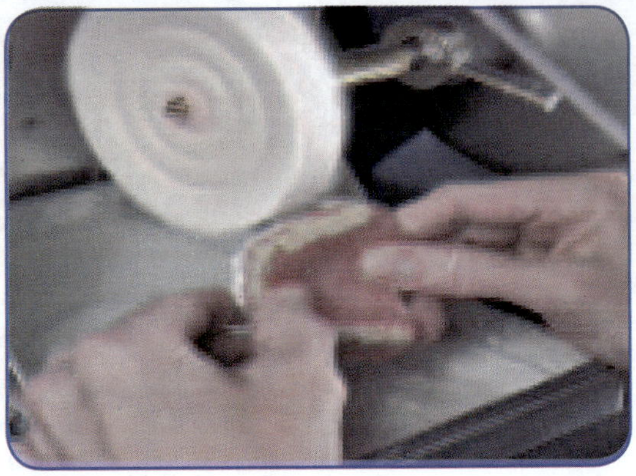

FINAL DENTURE

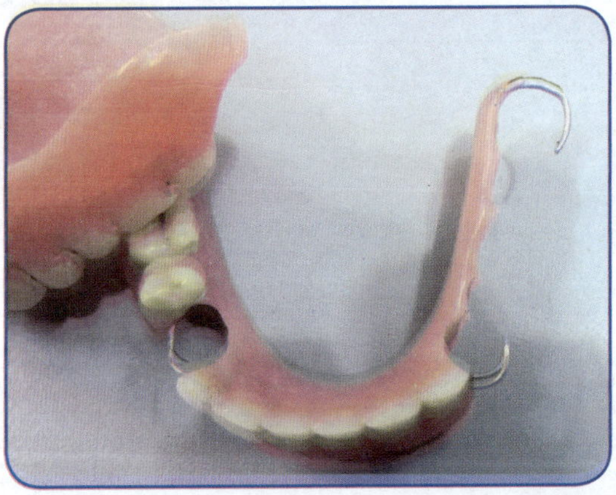

THIRD CLINICAL STEP

DENTURE INSERTION

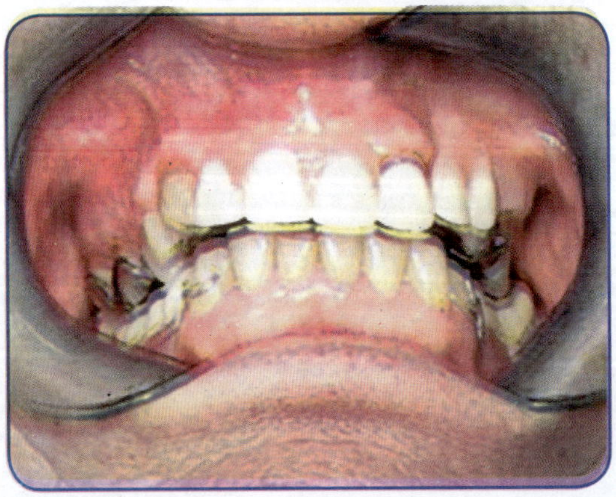

FIRST CLINICAL STEP

TRAY SELECTION

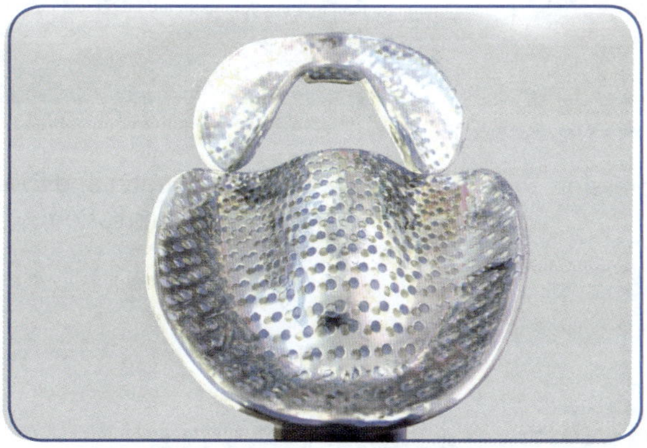

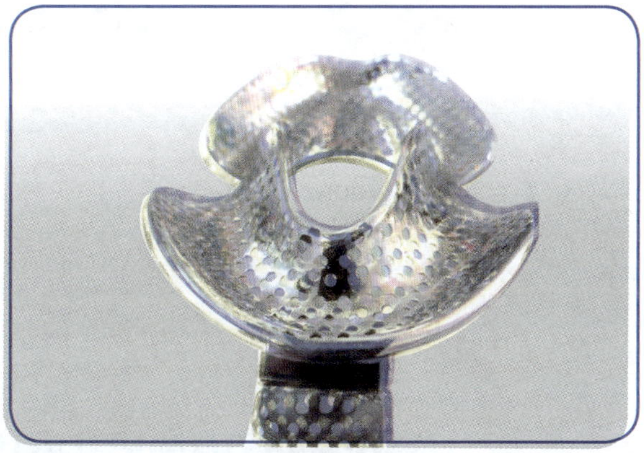

MANIPULATION OF IMPRESSION COMPOUND

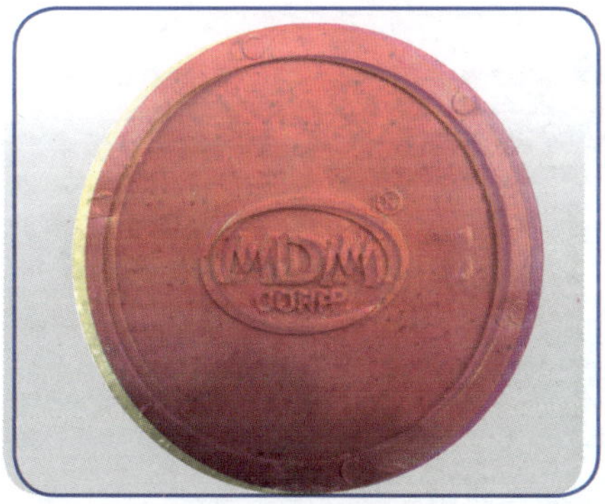

Dispensation
(Cake Form)

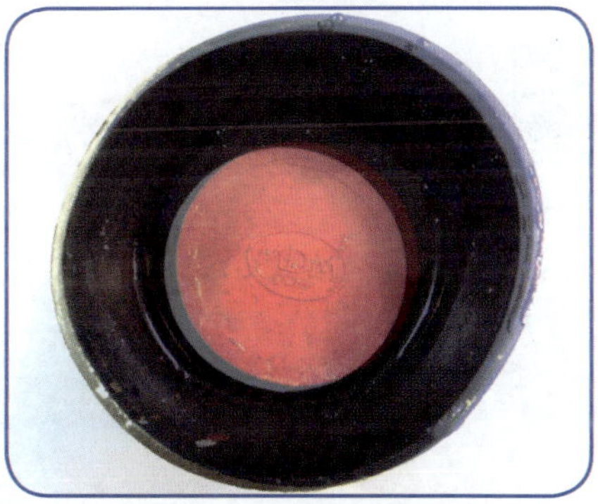

Impression Compound in
Warm Water (55-60°C)

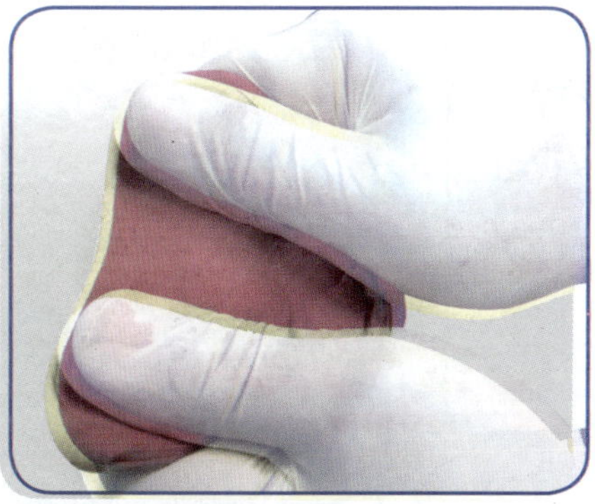

Kneading

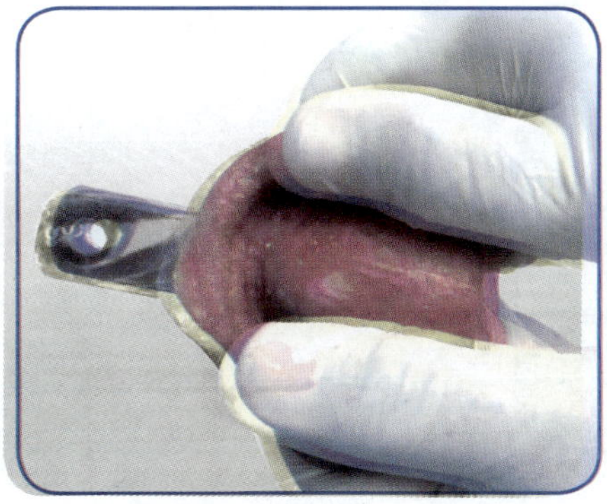

Loading of Impression Compound

INITIAL IMPRESSION

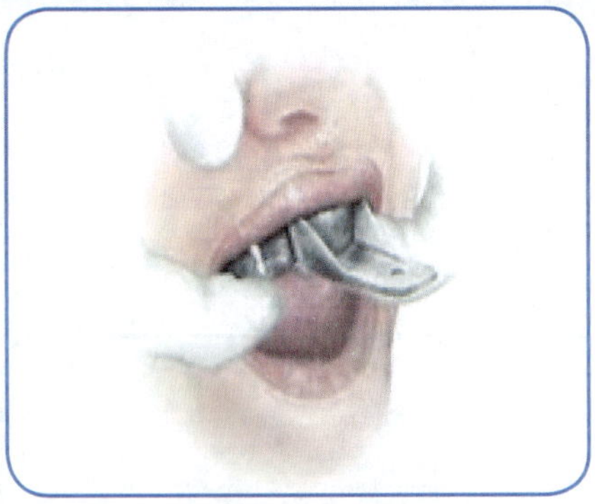

Tray Insertion

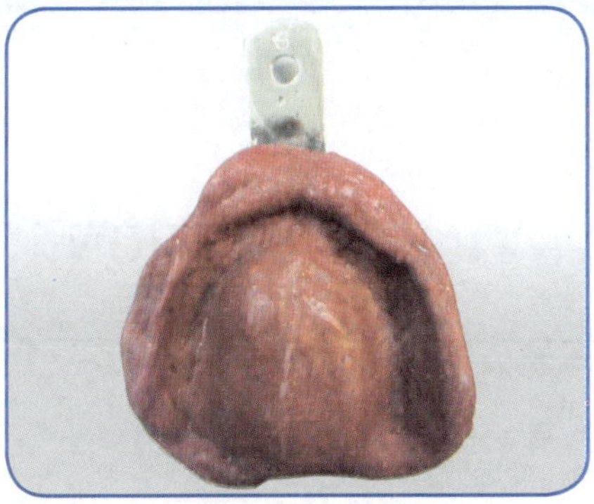

After Impression

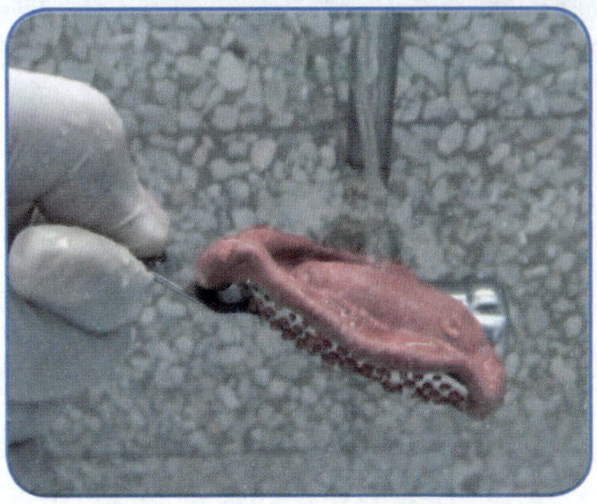

Wash With Tap Water and Disinfection of Impression

FIRST LABORATORY STEP

IMPRESSION POURING AND SEPARATION OF STOCK TRAY FROM MASTER CAST

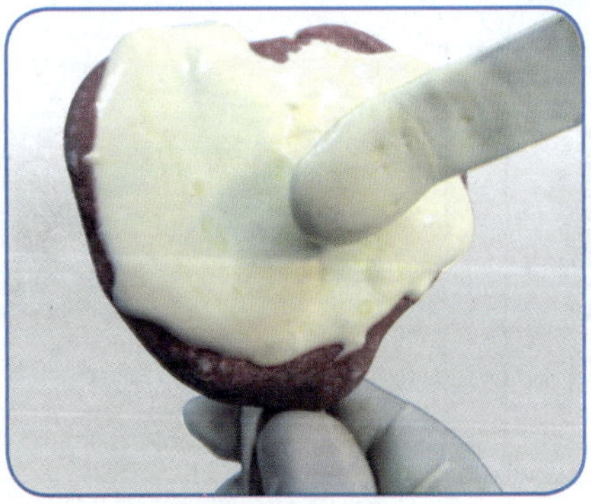

Impression Pouring

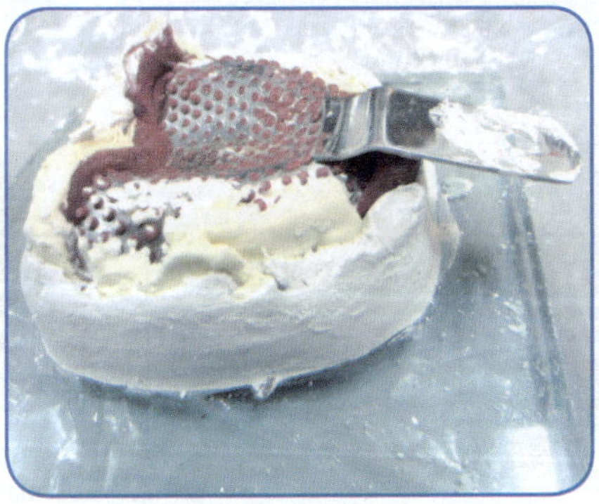

Base Formation

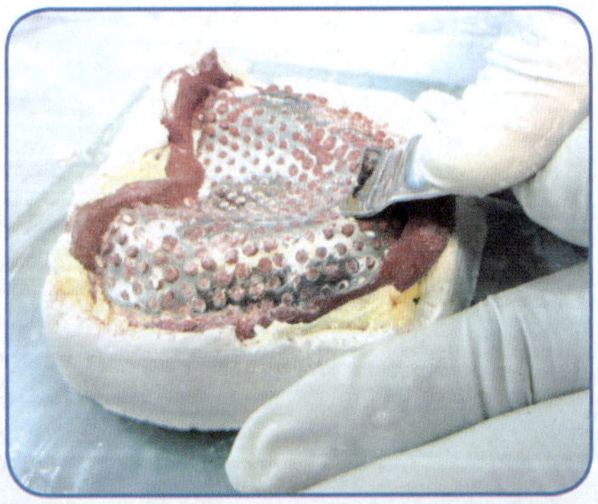

Hold Firmly During Removal of Impression Tray

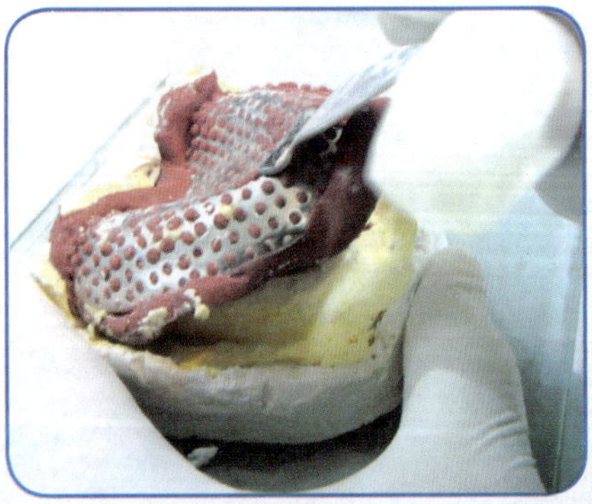

Removal of Impression Tray From the Cast

MAKING CUSTOM MADE TRAY BY SELF CURE ACRYLIC RESIN ON THE CAST

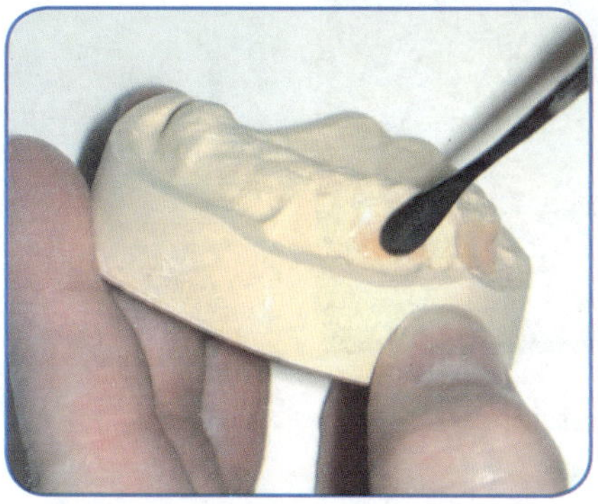

Blockout Under Cuts With Wax

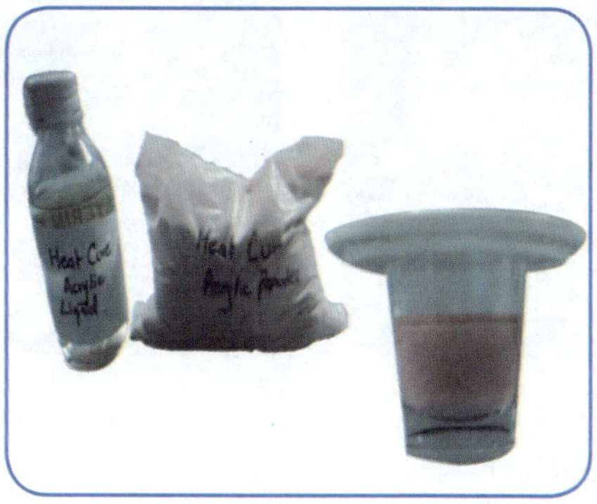

Self Cure Powder and Monomer Liquid

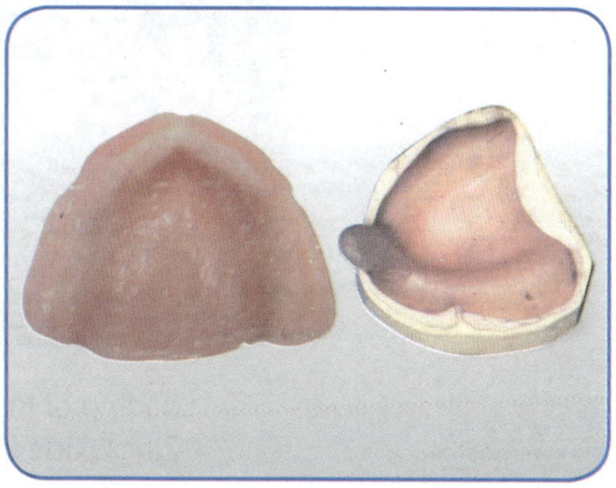

Self Cure Tray

SECOND CLINICAL STEP

APPLICATION OF GREEN STICK COMPOUND ON ACRYLIC TRAY

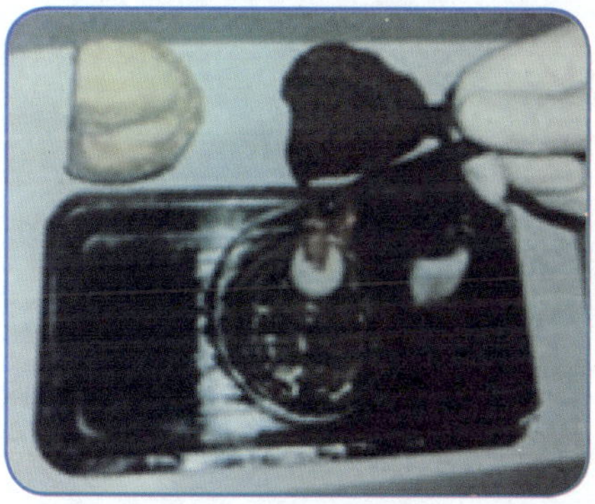

Manipulation of Stick Compound

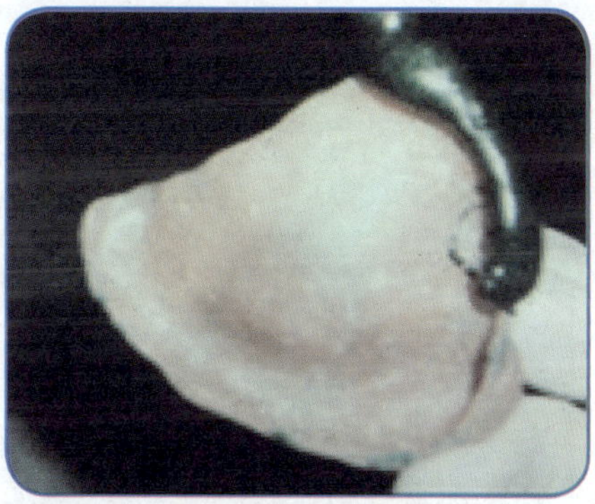

Loading of Green Stick Compound

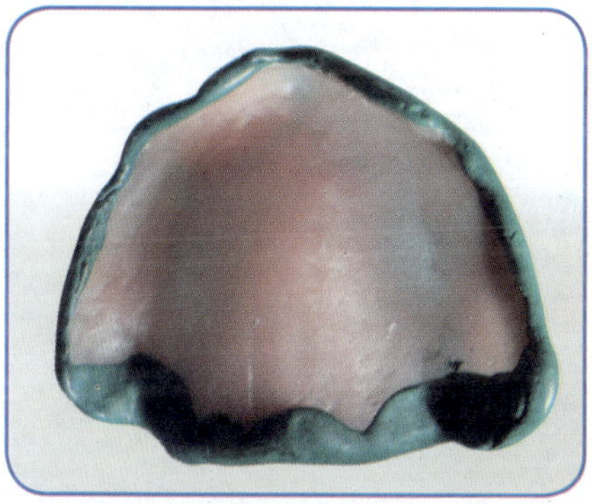

After Border Moulding

FINAL IMPRESSION OR WASH IMPRESSION

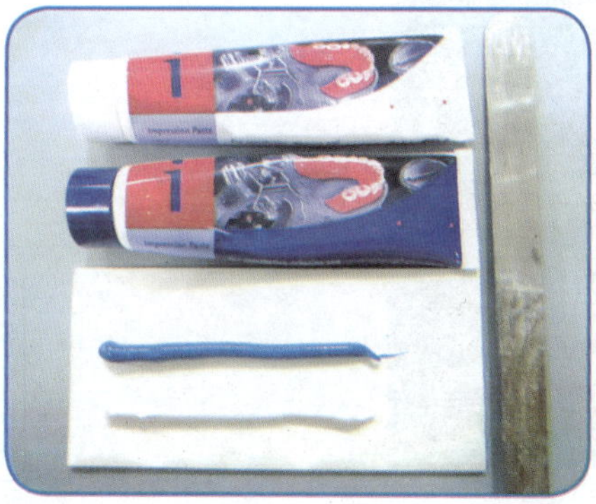

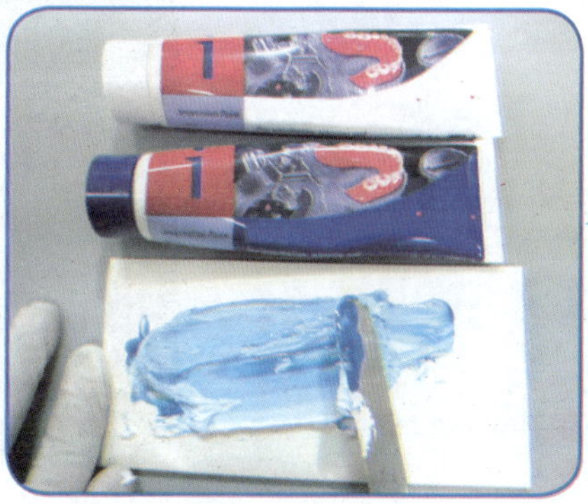

Mixing of Zinc Oxide Eugenol Impression Paste

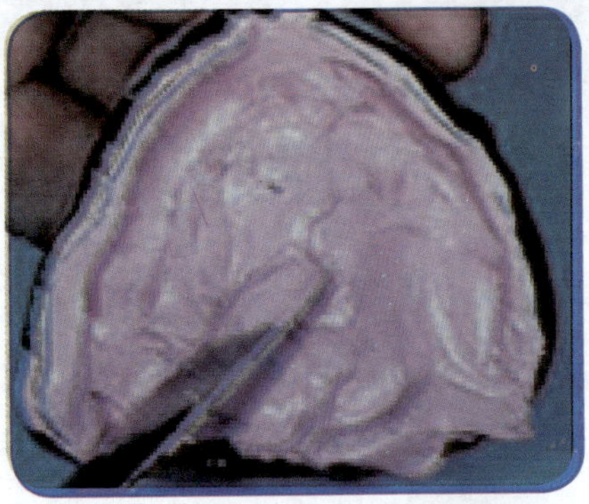

Loading of Impression With Zinc Oxide Eugenol Paste

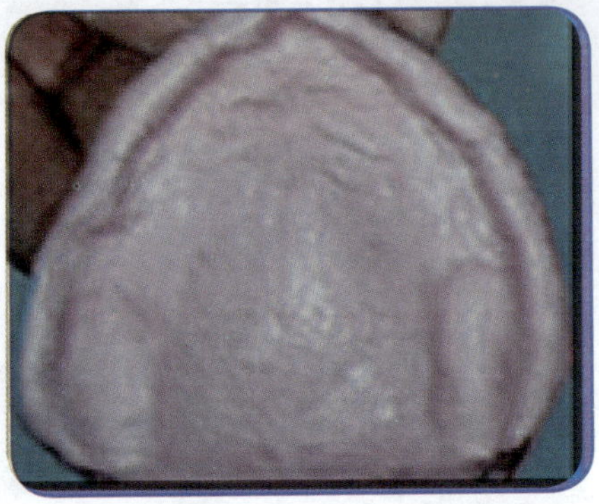

After Impression

SECOND LABORATORY STEP

POURING OF FINAL IMPRESSION FOR MAKING MASTER CAST

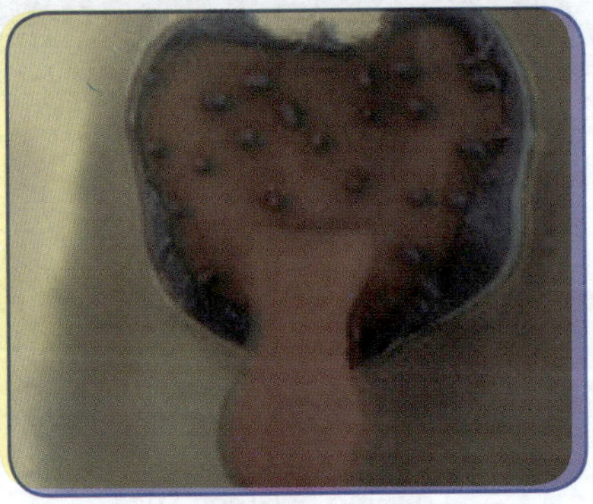

Pouring of Final Impression

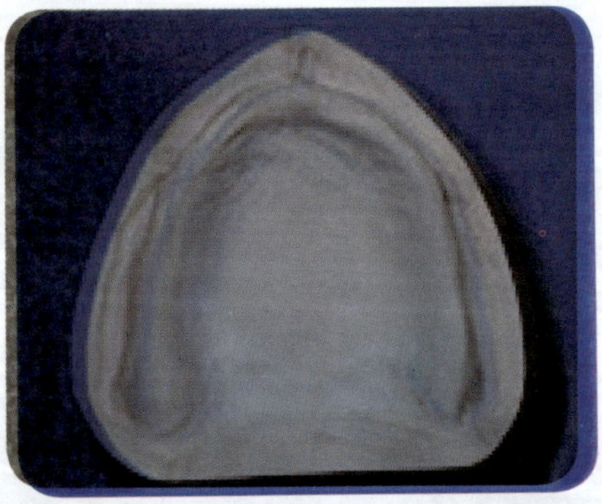

Master Cast

RECORD BASES AND OCCLUSAL RIMS FOR MAKING JAW RELATIONSHIP RECORDS

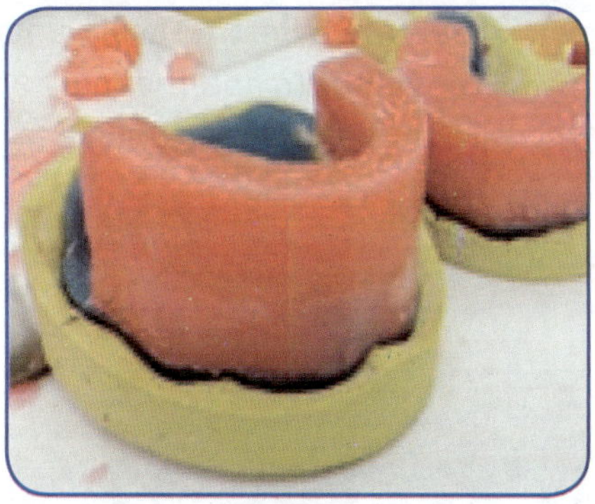

Record Rim

THIRD CLINICAL STEP

JAW RELATIONSHIP RECORD (MAXILLOMANDIBULAR RELATIONSHIP)

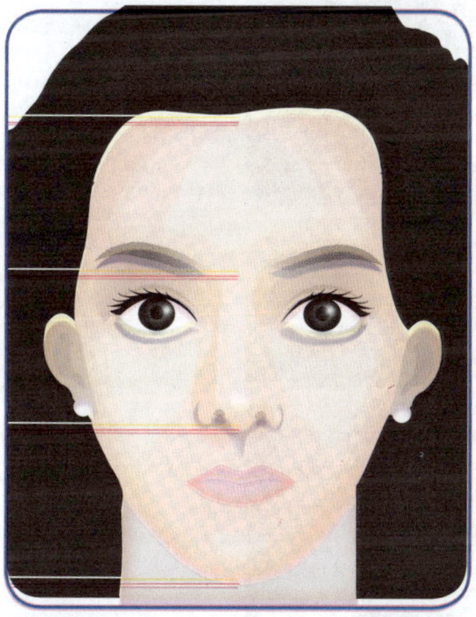

Proportioning the Face Clinically

VERTICAL RELATIONSHIP

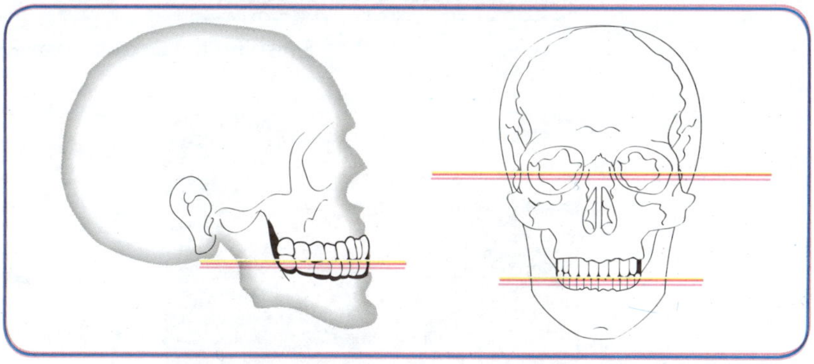

Ala-tragal Line

Interpupillary Line

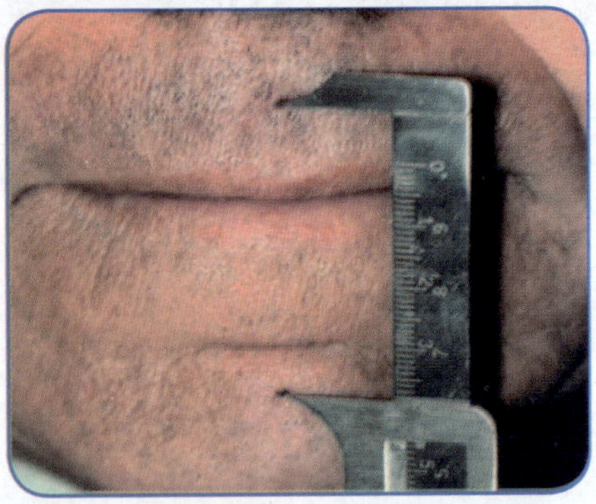

When the correct Rest Vertical Dimension (RVD) is established, the operator marks the philtrum and the most anterior point on the chin and measures the distance between the marks

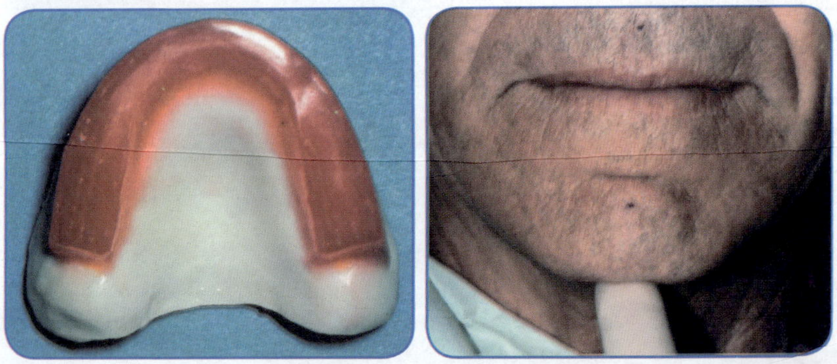

Checking the Occlusal Vertical Dimension (OVD) the superior-inferior relationship of the maxilla and the mandible when the teeth are situated in maximum intercuspation

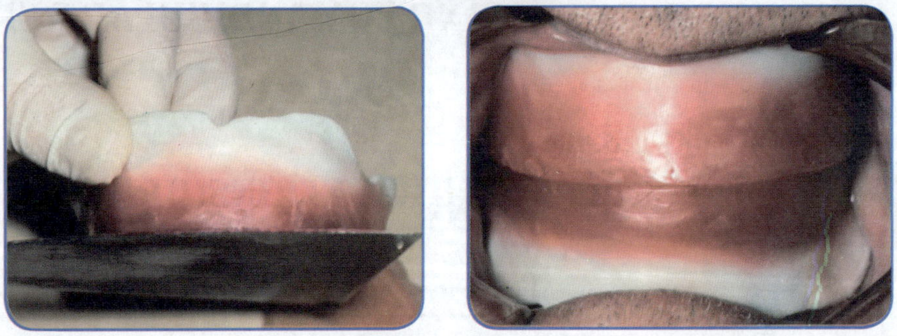

Finishing the Occlusal Wax Rims

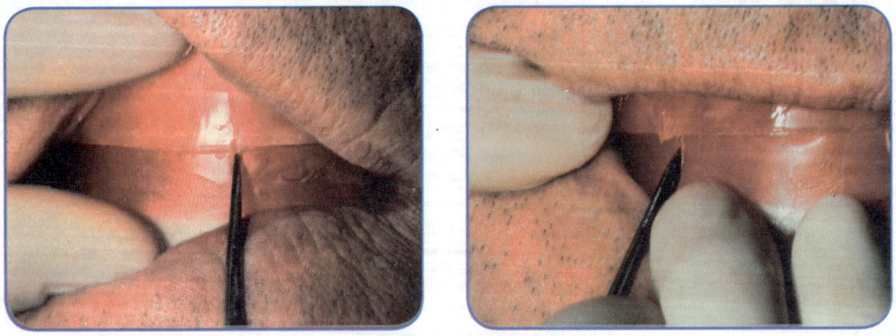

Centric Relation Registration

Place the occlusal rims in the patient's mouth and verify that both rims occlude evenly on closing. Close the patient's mouth into centric relation. Scribe a line on the right and left sides of the mandibular rim below the canine lines of the maxillary occlusal rim. This line will serve as a guide anteriorly when removing wax from the posterior side of the mandibular occlusal rim

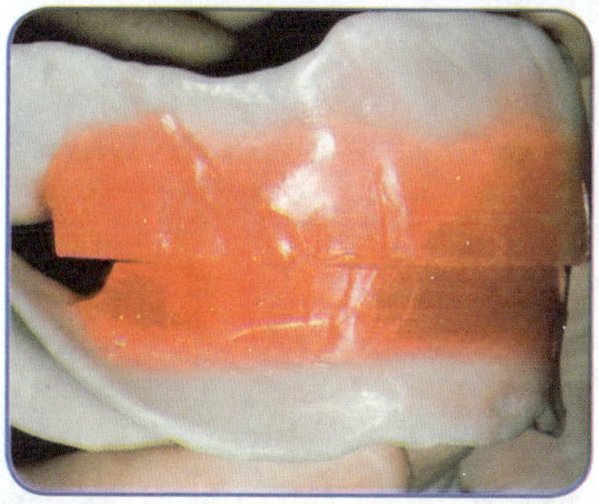

To Prevent Distorting the Record, a Heated Blade Should be Used to Seal it

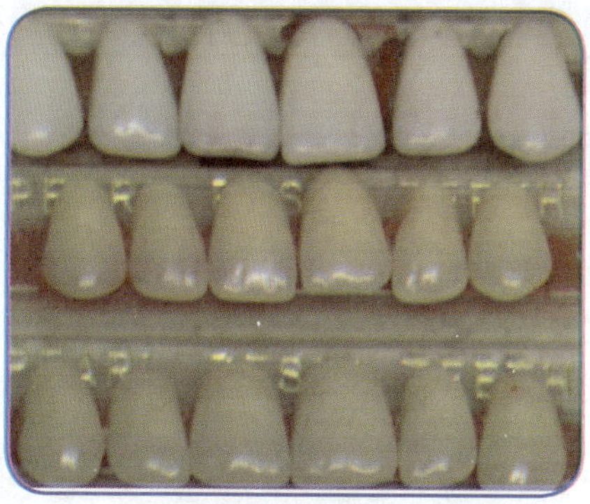

Selection of Artificial Teeth

THIRD LABORATORY STEP

ARTICULATION AND TEETH ARRANGEMENT

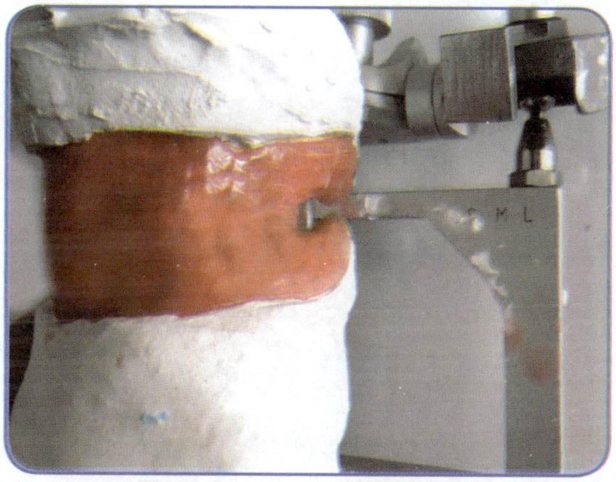

Seating the Cast on Articulator

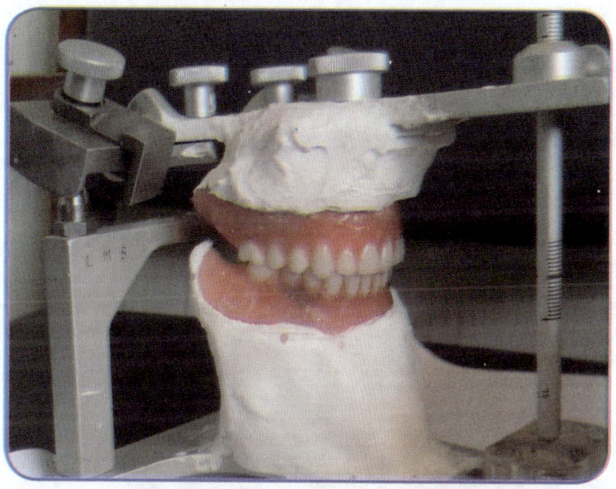

Setup of Teeth on Articulator

FOURTH CLINICAL STEP

DENTURE TRIAL

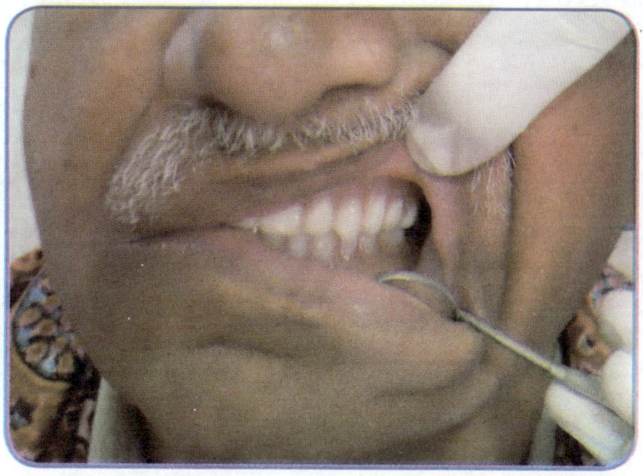

FOURTH LABORATORY STEP

DENTURE PROCESSING

FLASKING

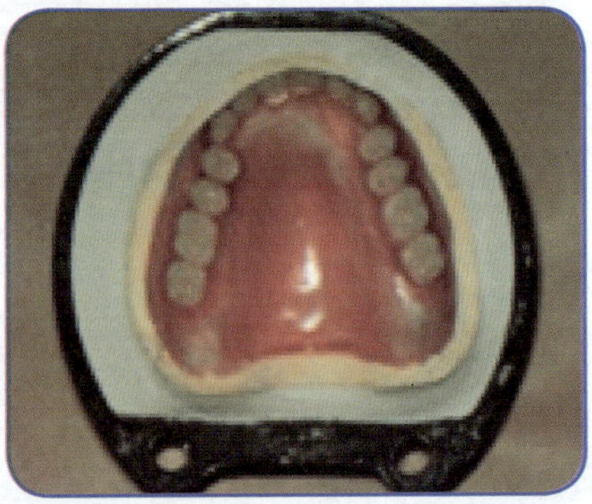

A

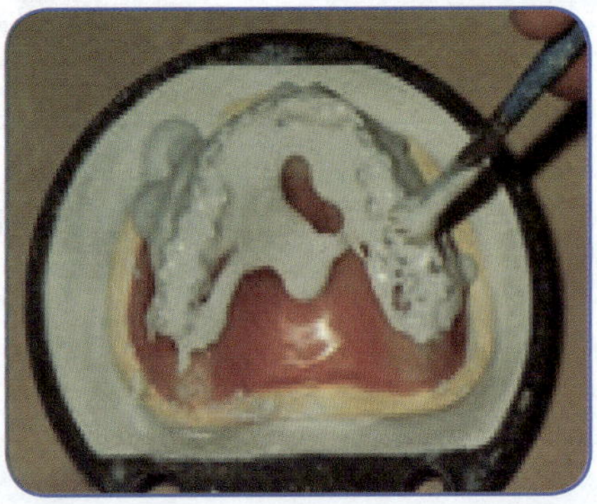

B

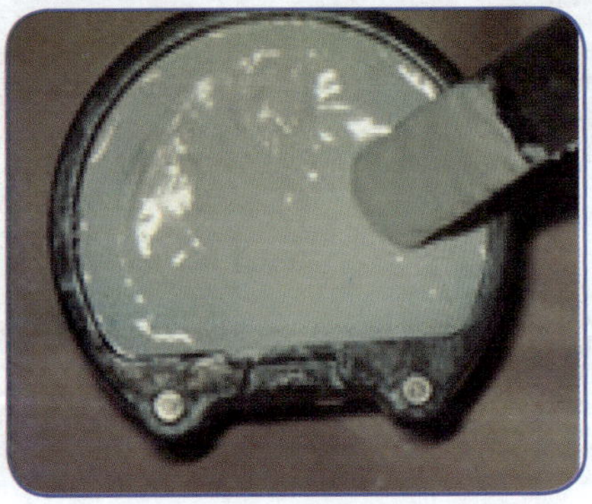

C

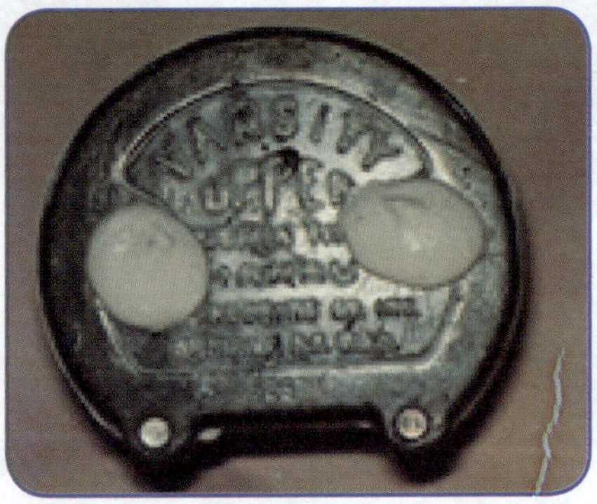

D

BOIL OUT WAX AND REMOVE RECORD BASES

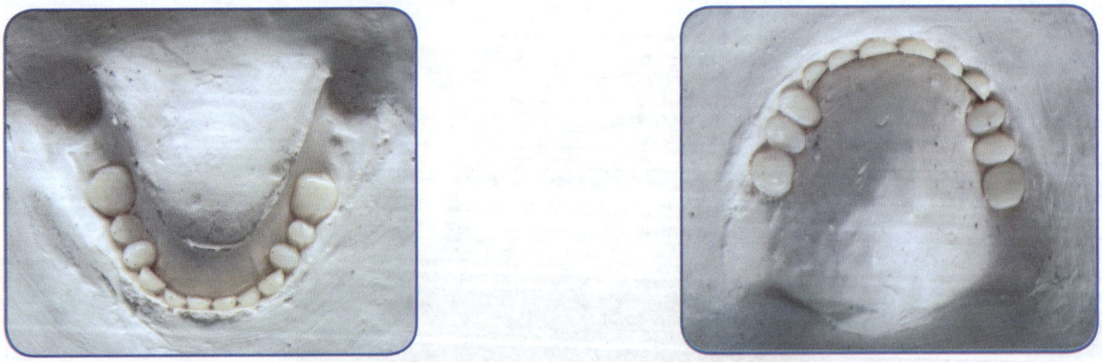

Teeth Trapped in Stone

PACKING AND CURING OF ACRYLIC RESIN

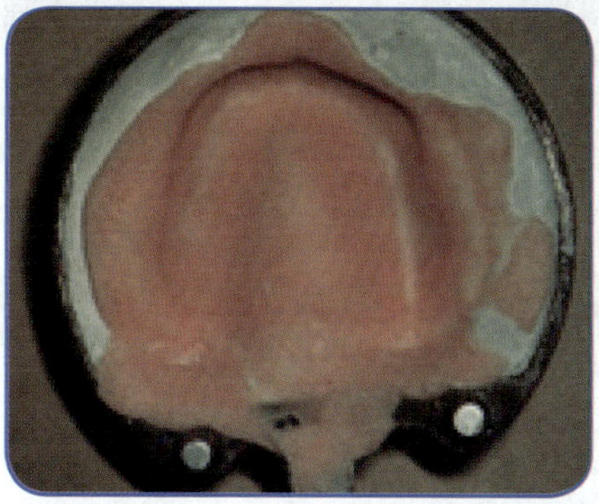

A

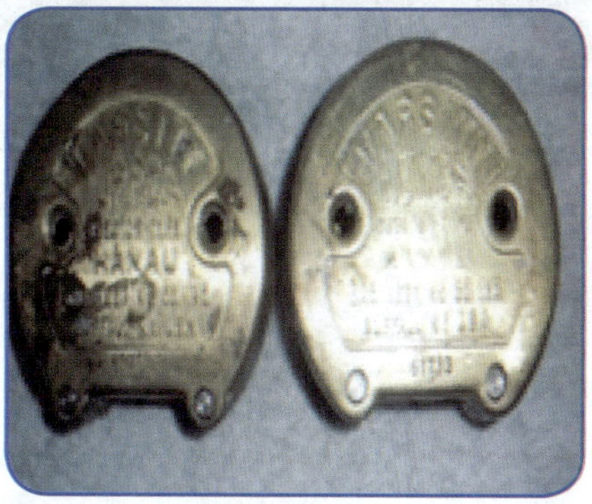

B

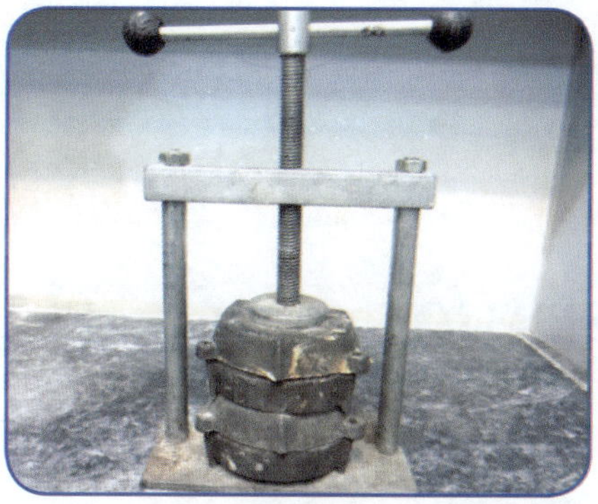

C

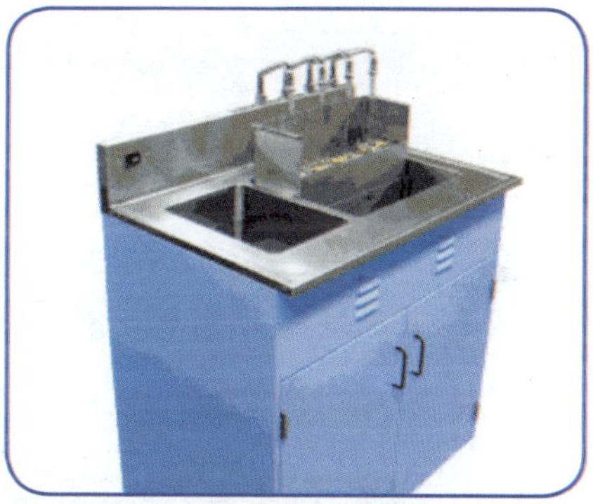

D

REMOVE FROM CAST

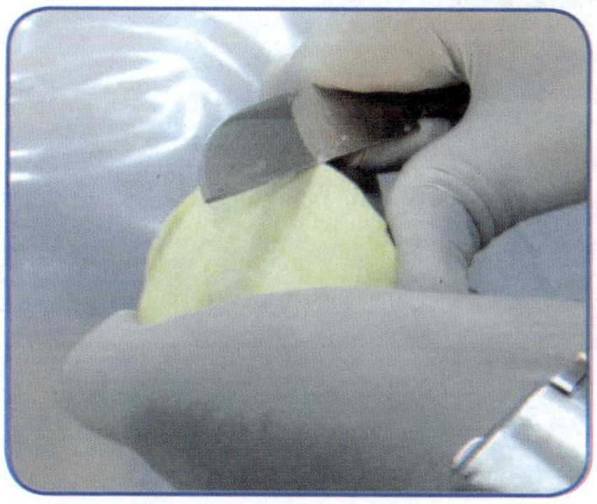

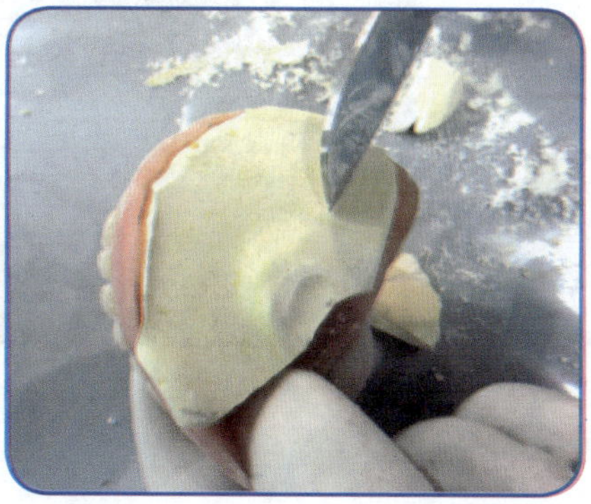

FINISHING AND POLISHING

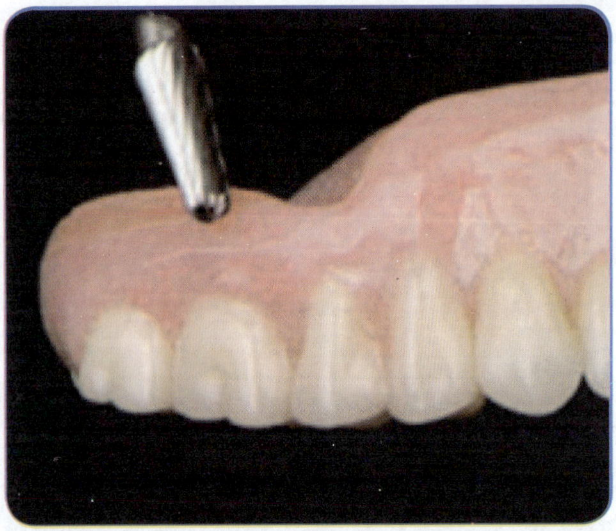

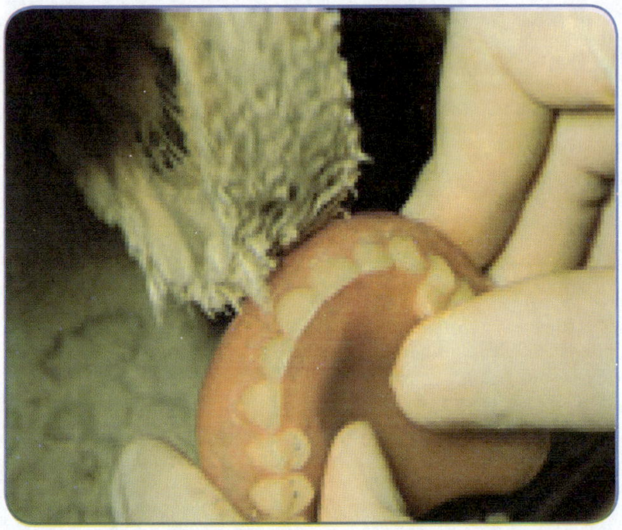

FIFTH CLINICAL STEP

DENTURE INSERTION

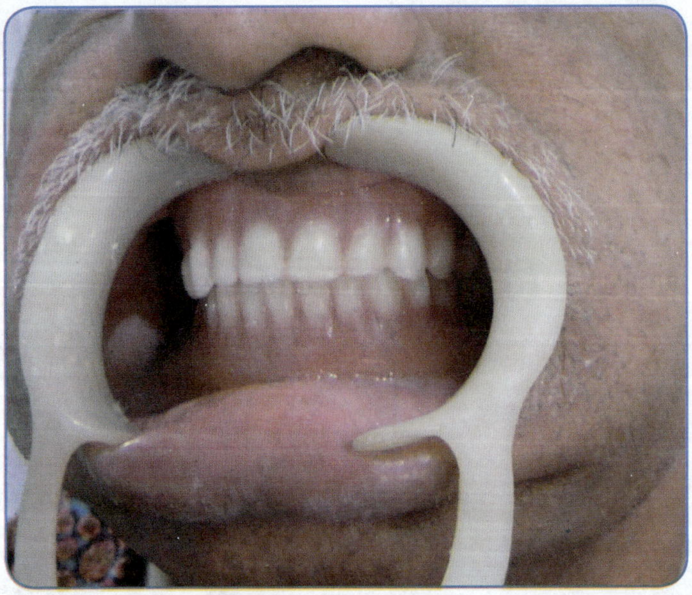

PHOTOGRAPHIC PRESENTATION OF IMPRESSIONS, WAXES, DIRECT AND INDIRECT RESTORATIONS

14
PRACTICAL

DISPENSING, MIXING, MANIPULATION AND RESTORATION

ALGINATE
(ELASTIC IMPRESSION MATERIAL)

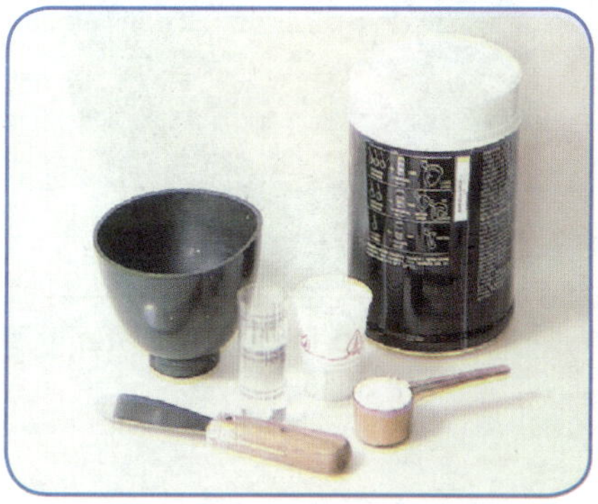

Dispensing

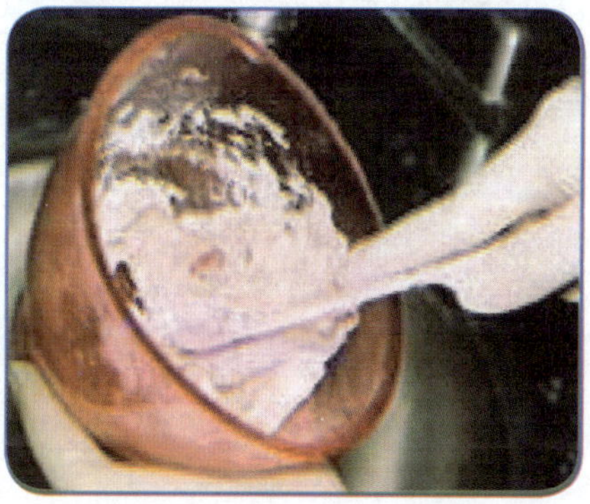

Mixing

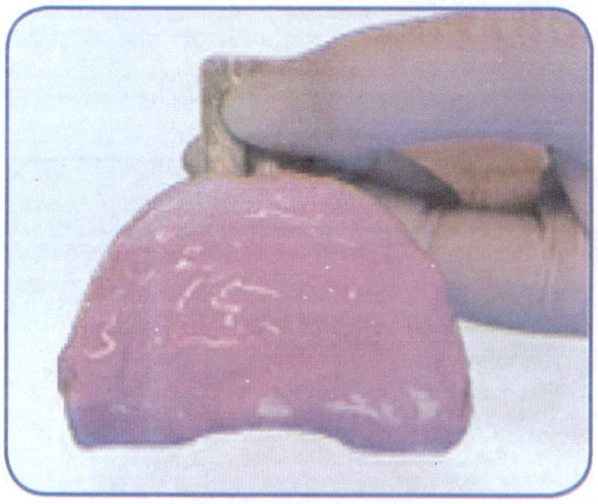

Alginate Impression on Stock Tray

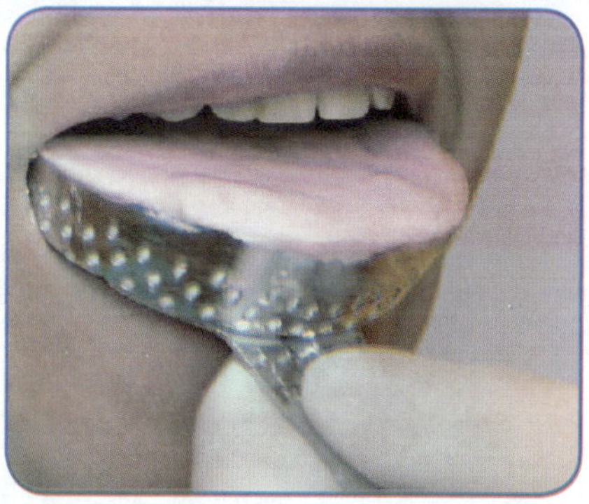

Impression Taking

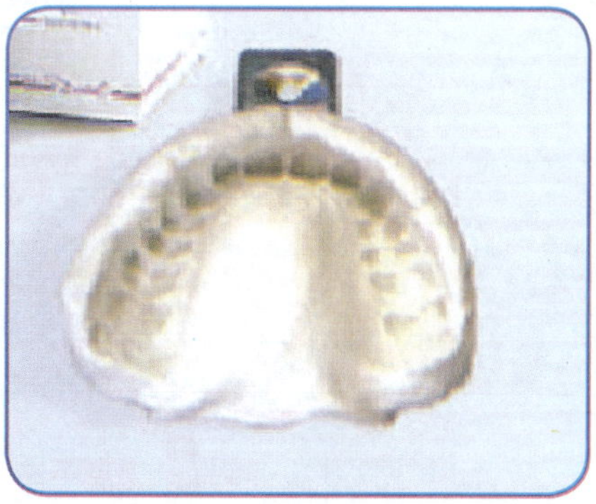

After Impression

Photographic Presentation

IMPRESSION COMPOUND CAKE/SHEET FORM (NON ELASTIC IMPRESSION MATERIAL)

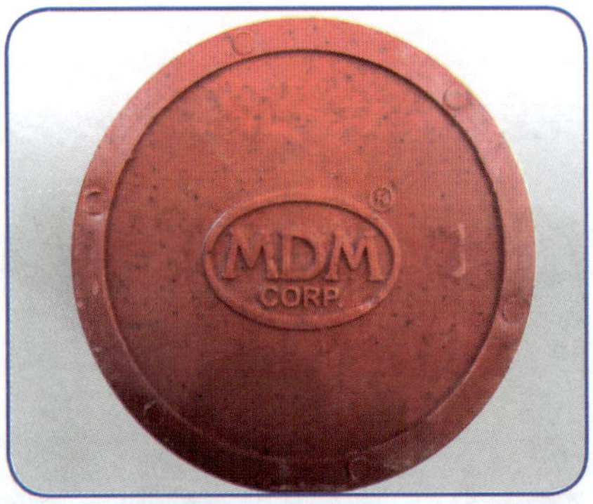

Dispensing

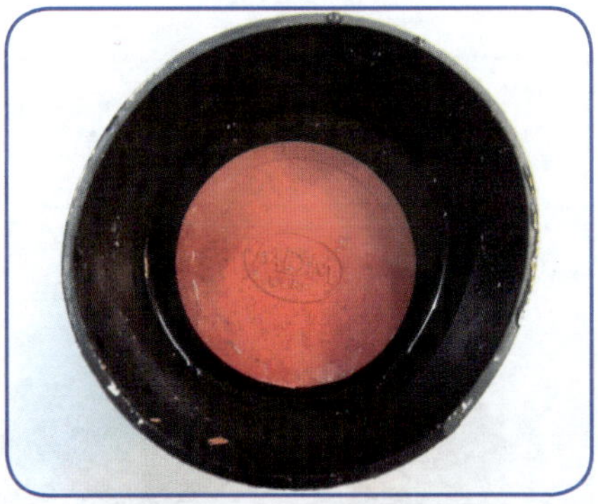

Imp. Compo. in a Warm Water at 55-60°C

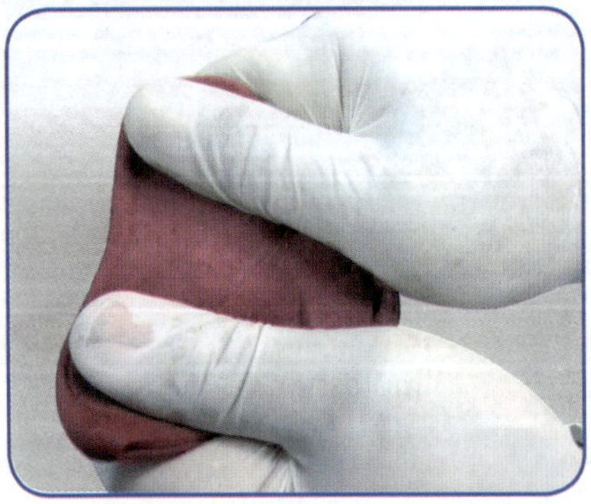

Kneading

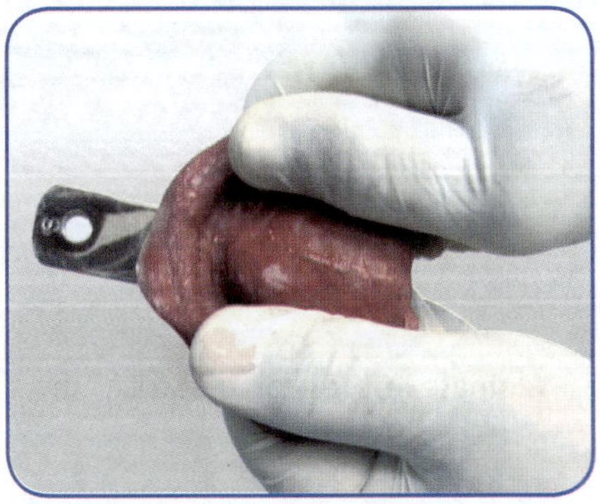

Impression Loading on Tray

Photographic Presentation

IMPRESSION COMPOUND STICK FORM (NON ELASTIC IMPRESSION MATERIAL)

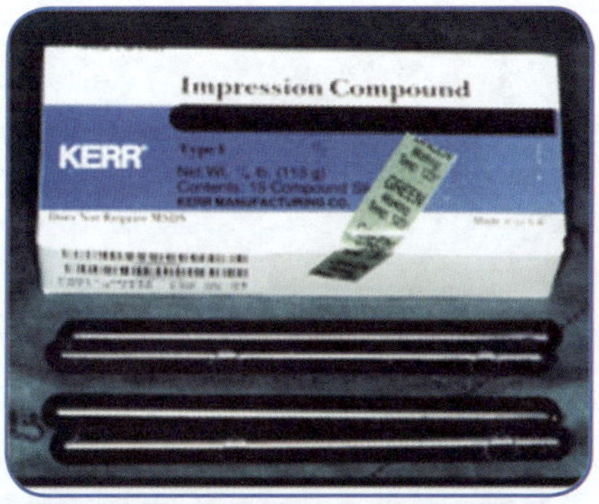

Dispensing

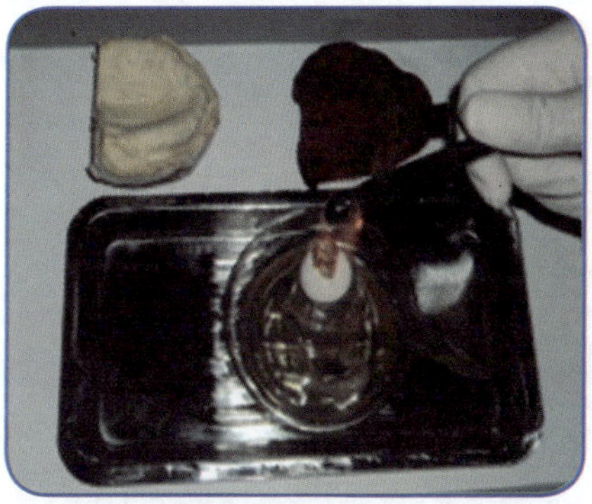

Manipulation of Impression (Stick Form)

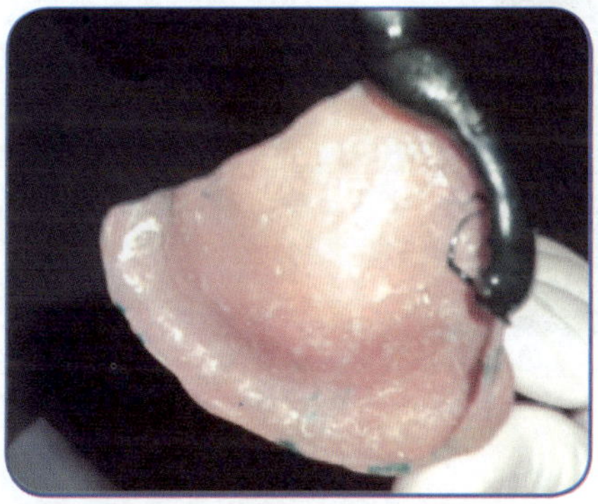

Loading of Stick Form Impression on Custom Made Tray

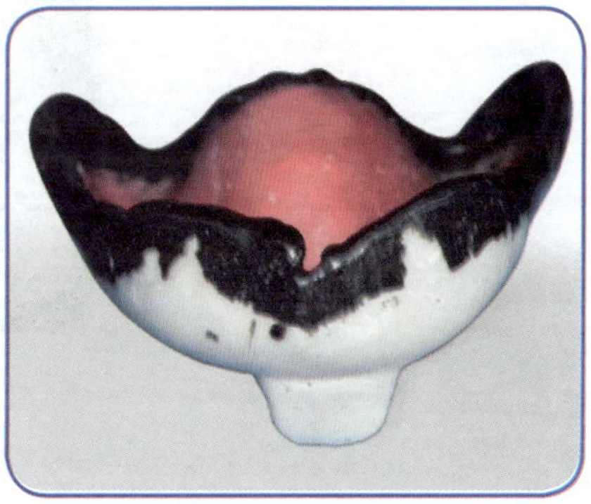

After Border Molding

Photographic Presentation

ZINC OXIDE EUGENOL IMPRESSION MATERIAL (NON ELASTIC IMPRESSION MATERIAL)

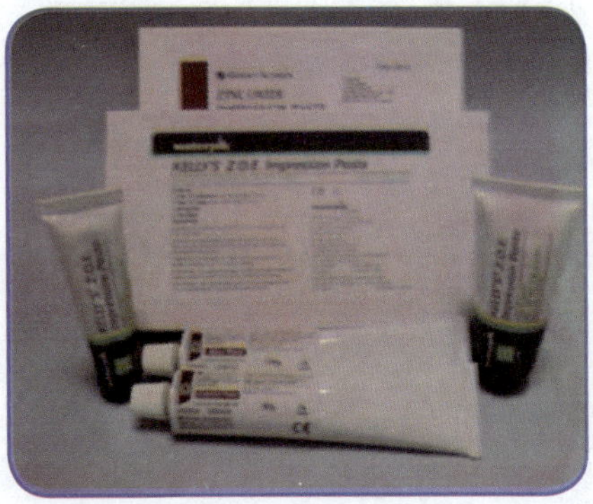

Dispensing in Tubes
(Base and Catalyst)

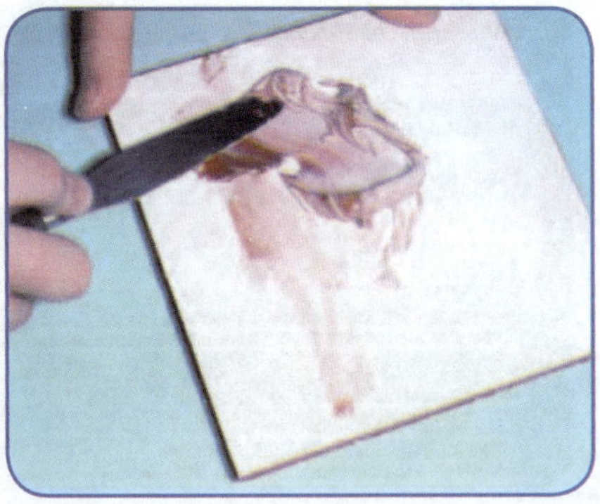

Mixing of Impression on Paper Pad

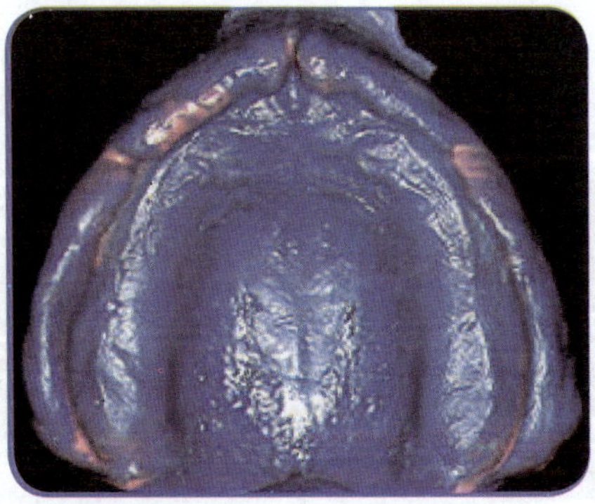

After Final Impression
(Wash Impression)

Photographic Presentation

DENTAL WAXES

PATTERN WAXES

i. INLAY WAX

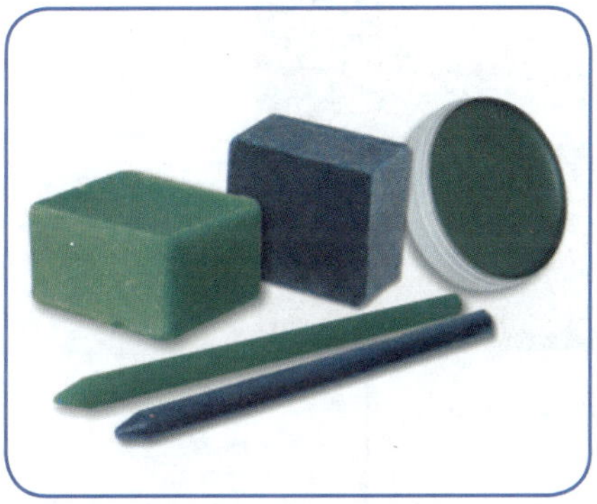

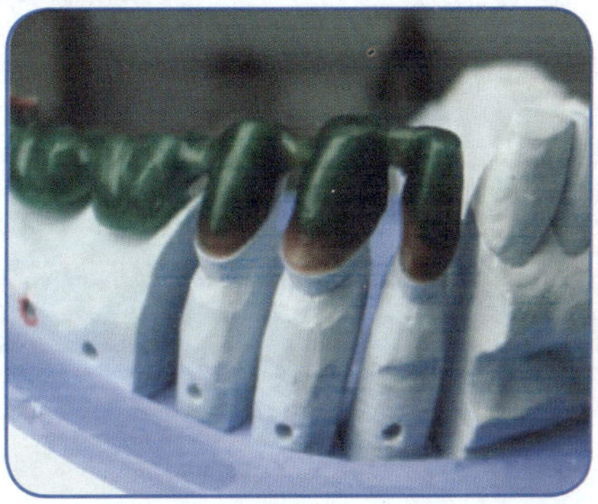

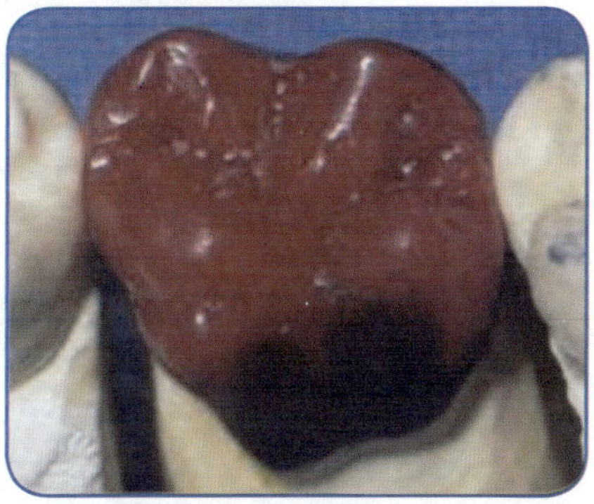

SPRUE WAX

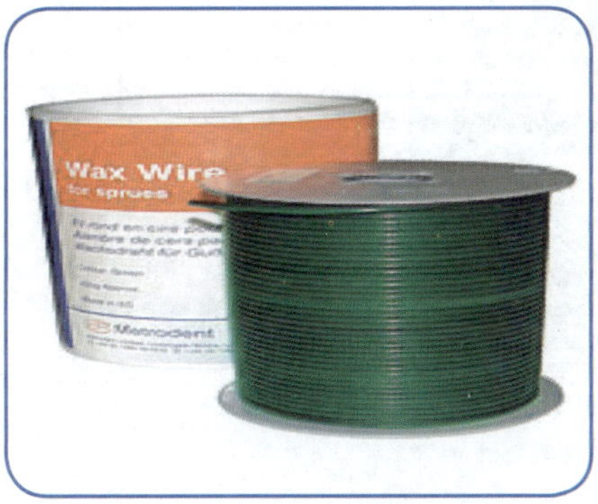

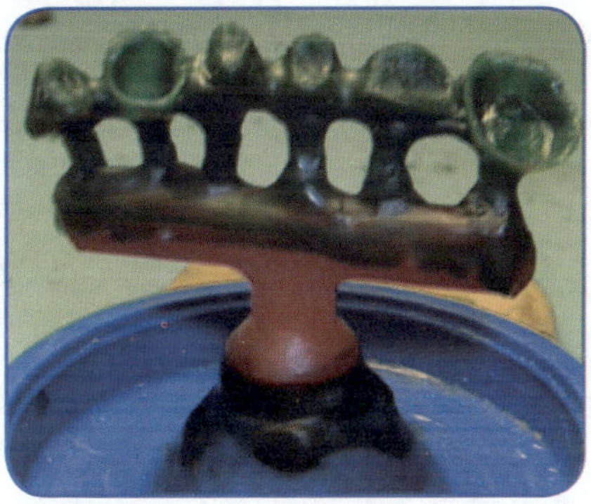

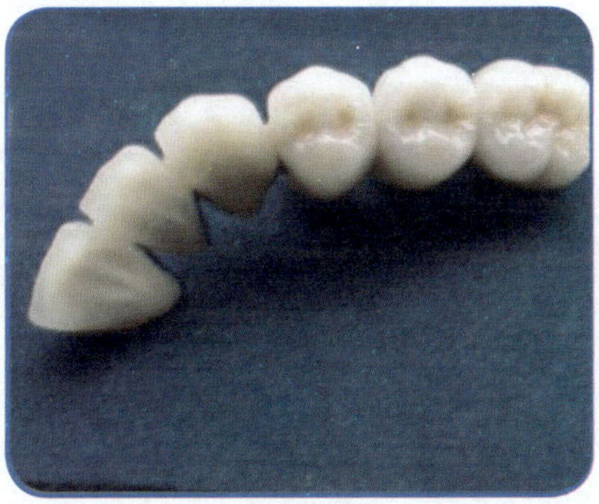

Porcelain Fused to Metal

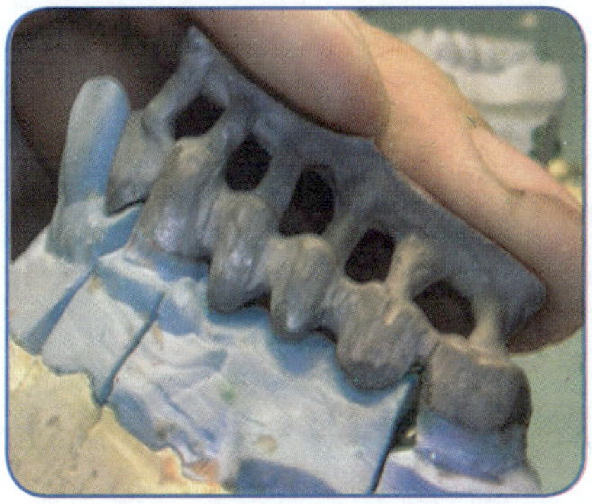

Metal Frame Work for Porcelain

CASTING WAX

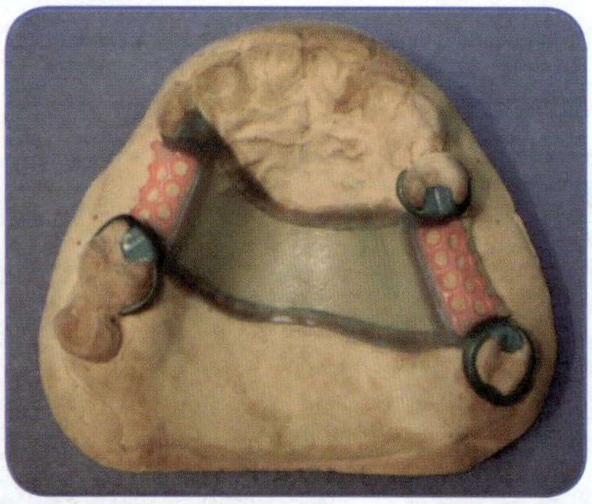

Wax up

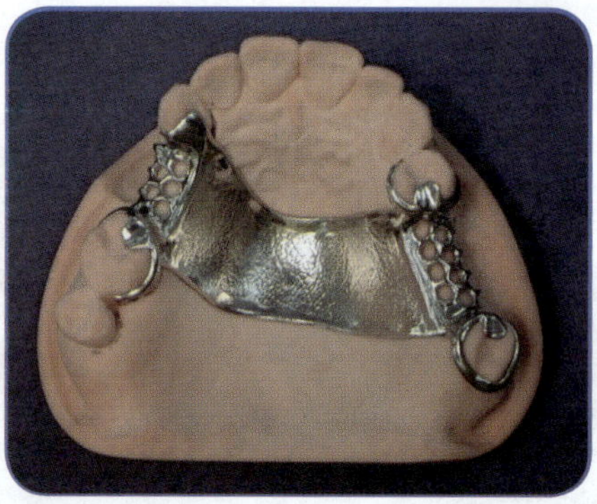

Metal Frame Work

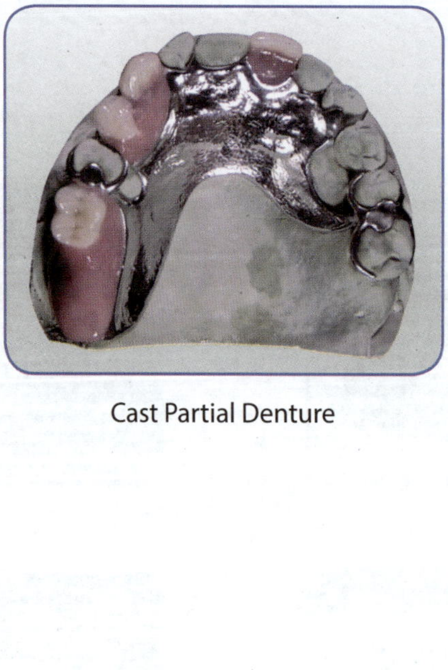

Cast Partial Denture

Photographic Presentation

ii. MODELLING/BASE PLATE WAX

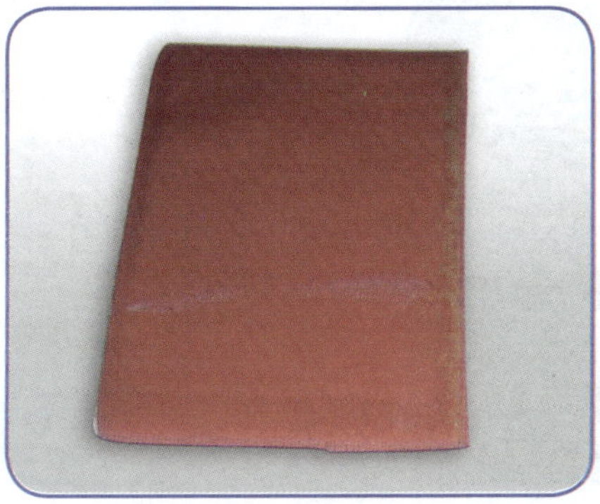

Wax Sheet

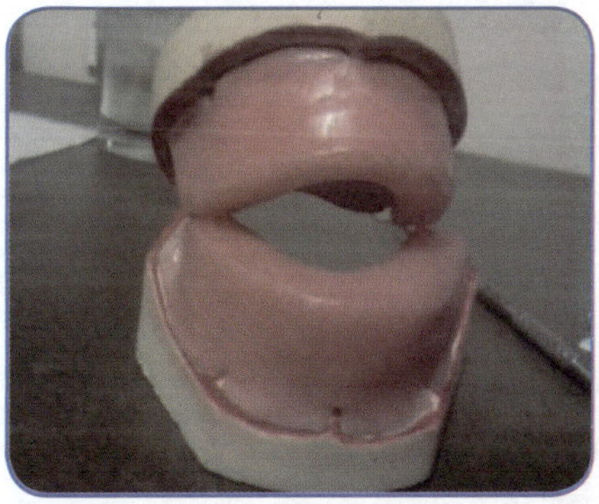

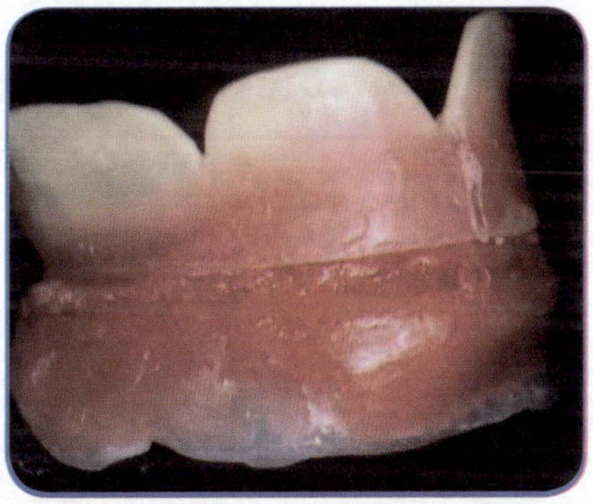

Base Plate Wax

BOXING WAX

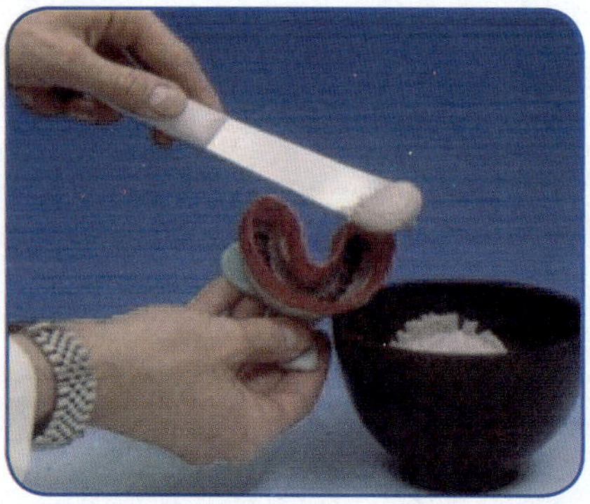

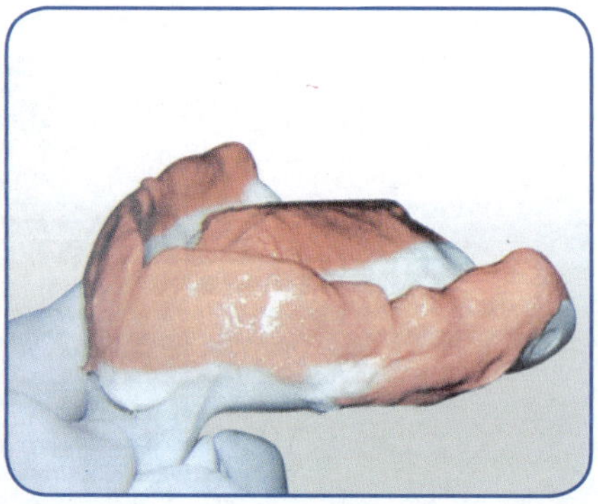

CARDING WAX

Photographic Presentation

UTILITY WAX

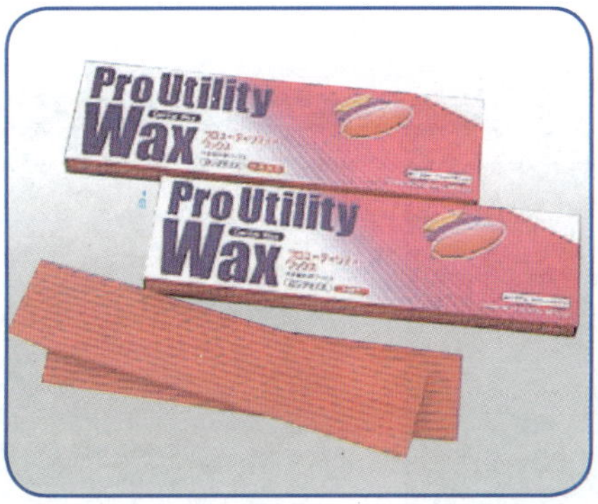

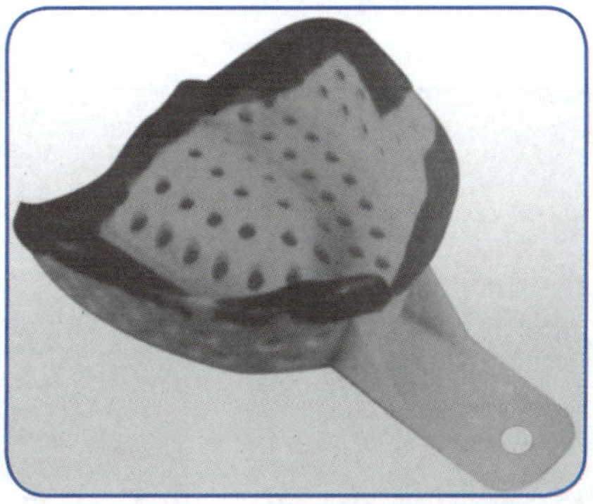

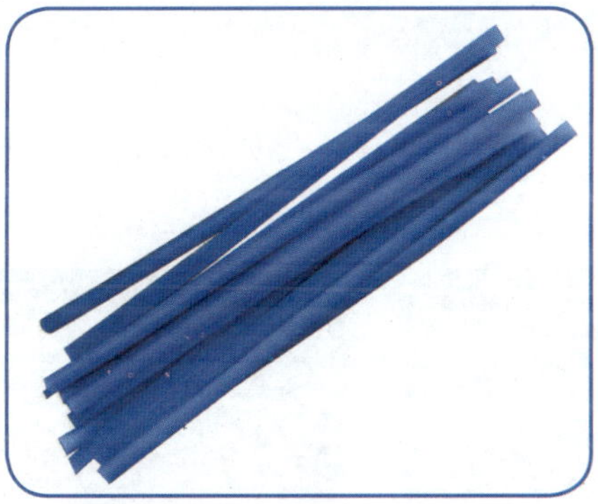

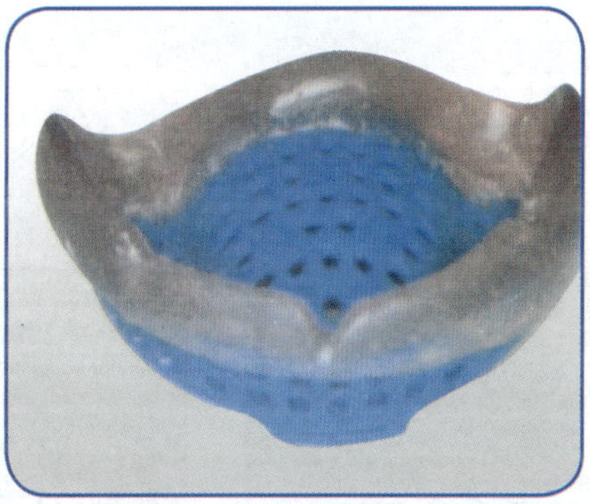

STICKY WAX

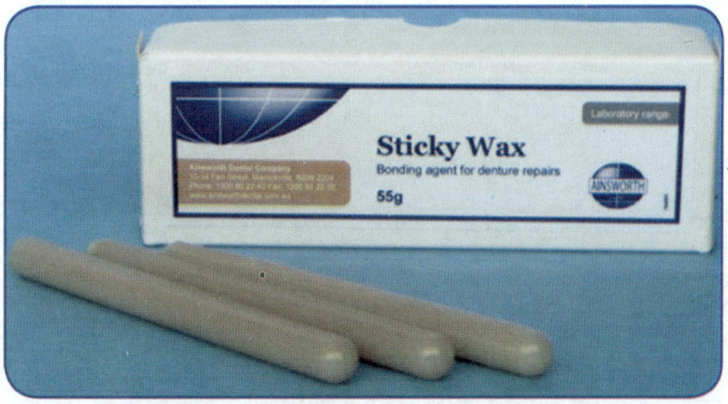

Photographic Presentation

PHYSICAL STAGES OF POLYMERISATION (ACRYLIC RESIN)

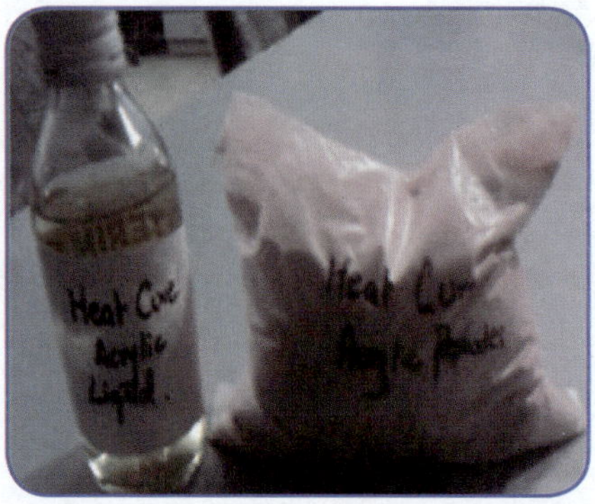

Acrylic Powder and Liquid Monomer

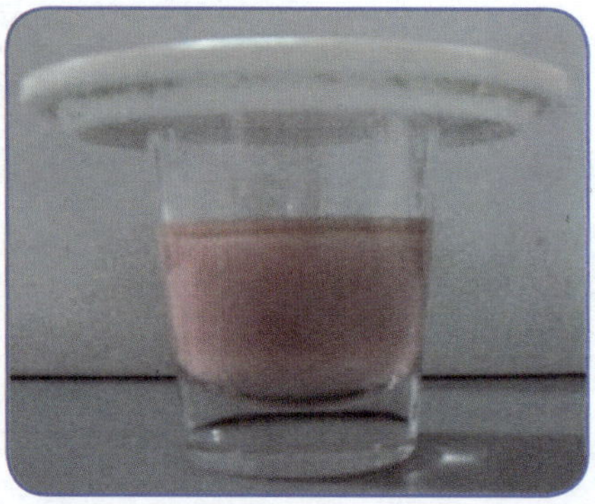

Mixing of Powder and Liquid

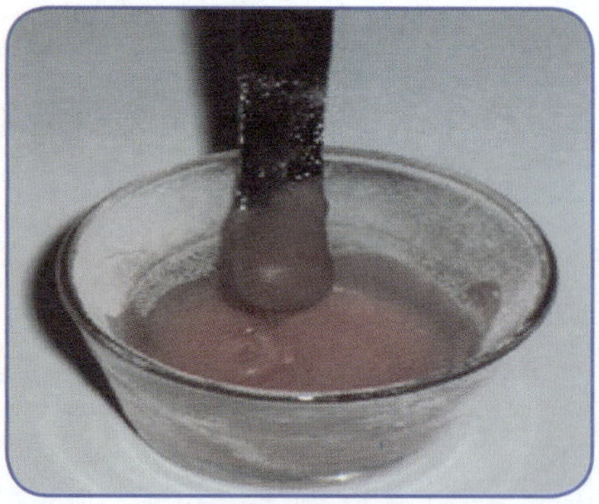

Sandy Phase

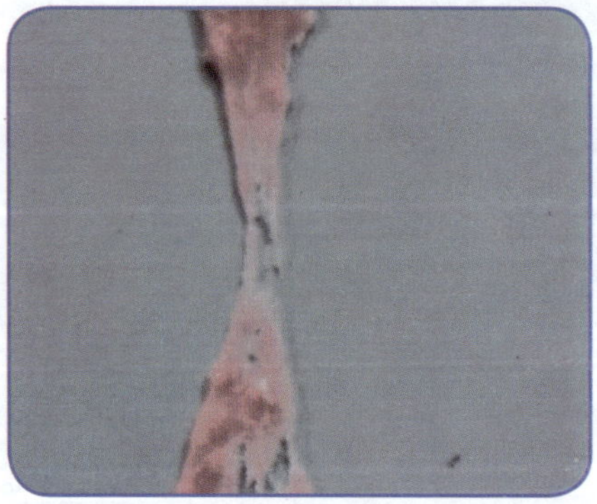

Stringy Phase

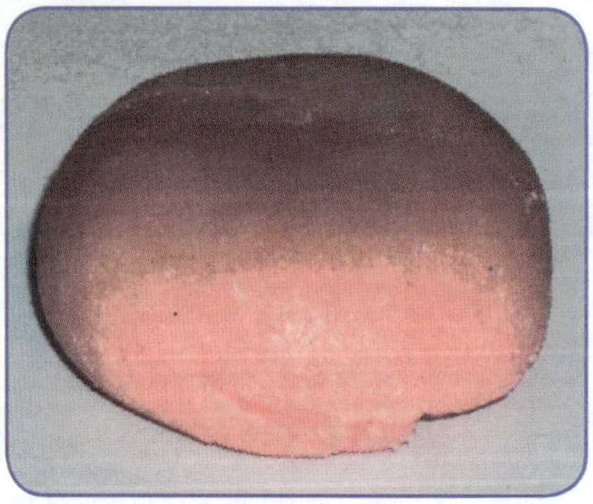

Doughy Phase

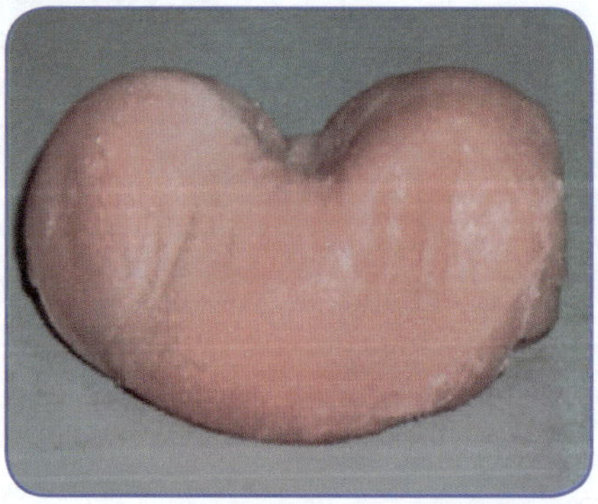

Rubbery Phase

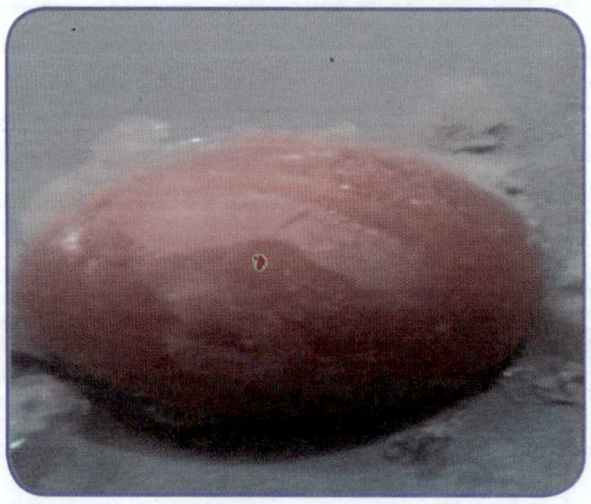

Hard / Stiff Phase

Photographic Presentation

DIRECT RESTORATIVE MATERIALS (TOOTH COLORED)

DISPENSING OF GLASS IONOMER CEMENT

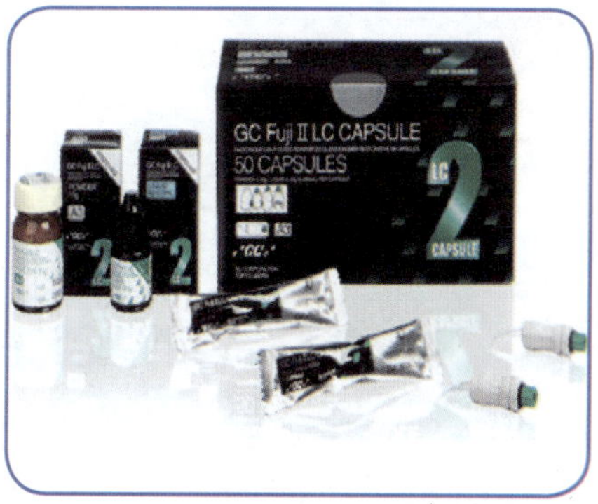

Dispensing (P/L)

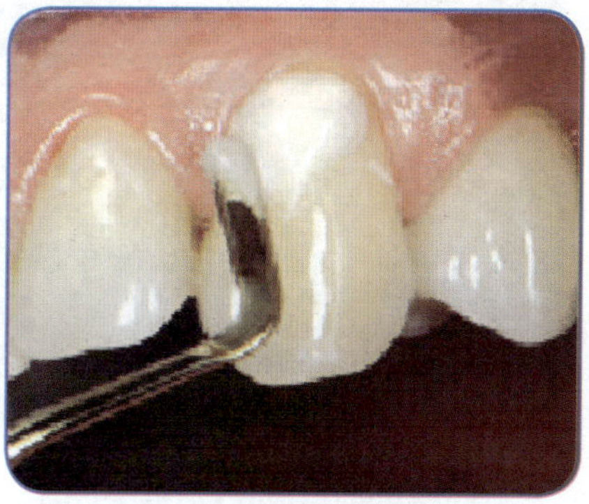

Restoration of Glass Ionomer Cement

LIGHT CURE COMPOSITE RESTORATIVE MATERIAL

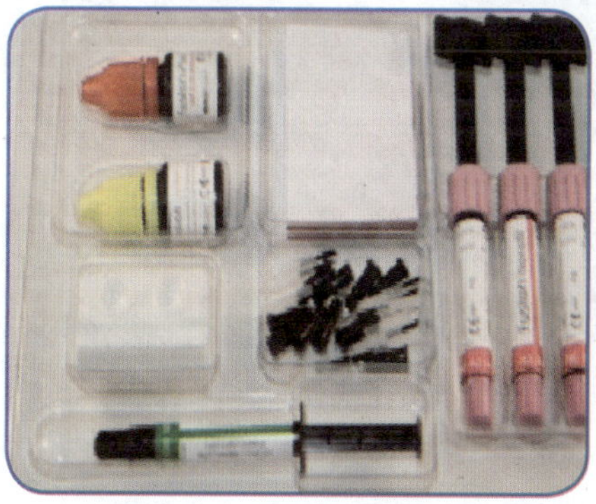

Dispensing (Composite Kit)

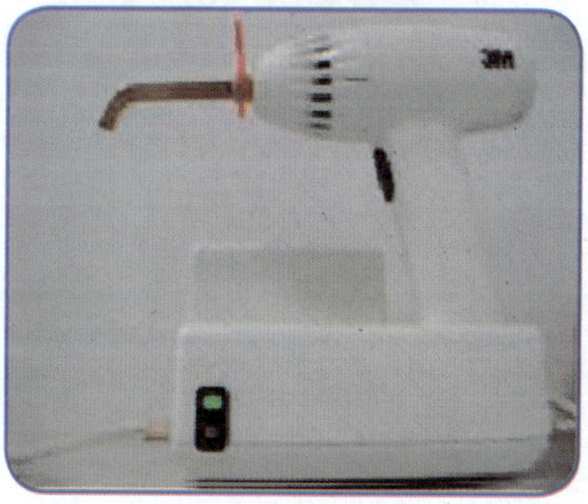

Light Curing Unit

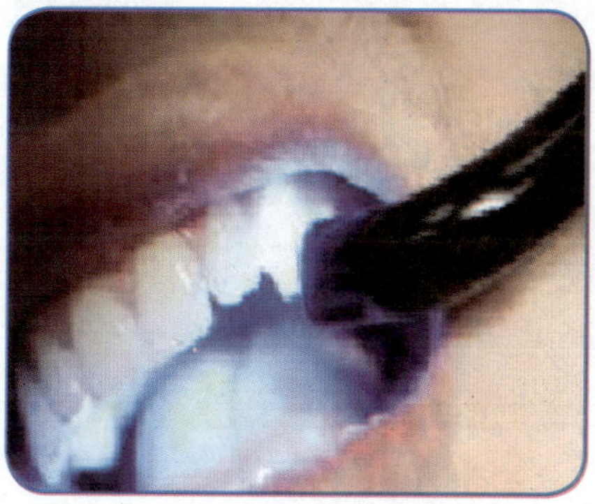

Curing With Light Source

Photographic Presentation

DENTAL AMALGAM
(DIRECT METALLIC RESTORATION)

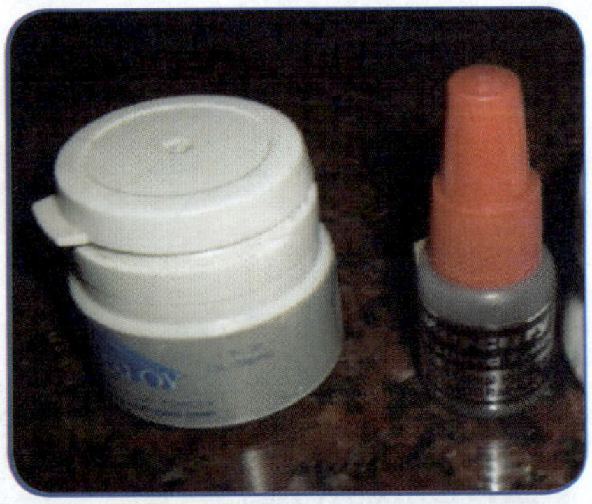

Hand Mixing (Alloy / Mercury)

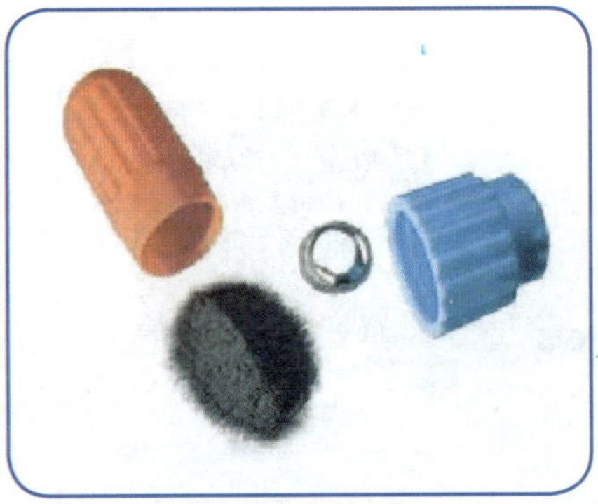

Encapsulated Form

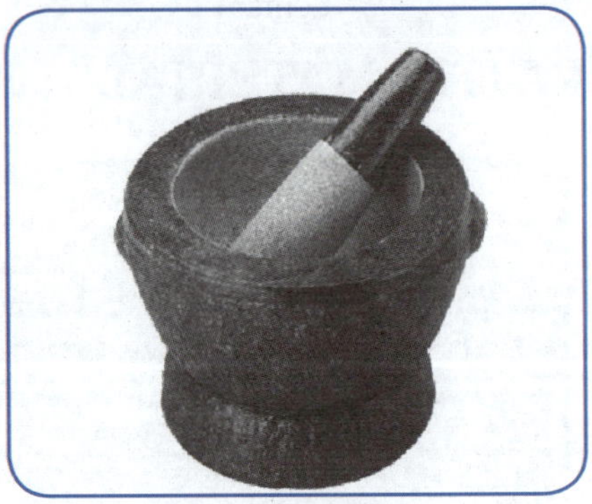

Mortar and Pestle
(Hand Mixing)

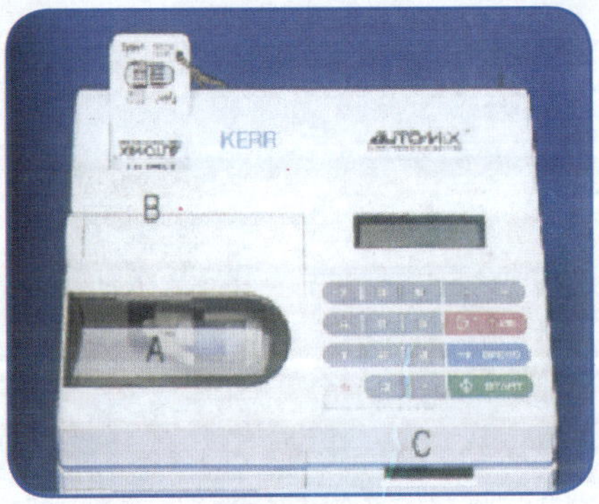

Amalgamator
(Mechanical Mixing)

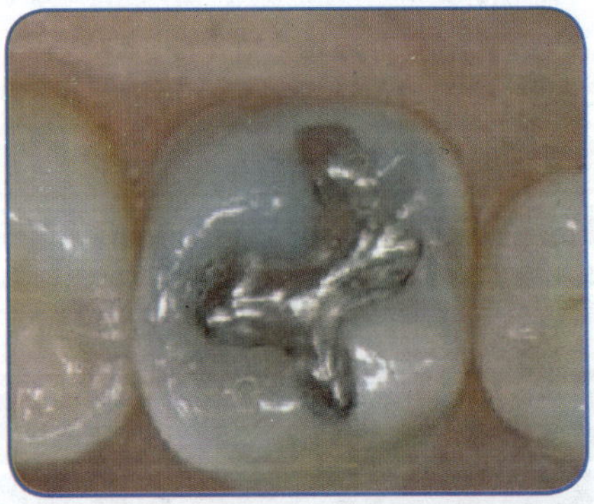

Dental Amalgam Restoration

Photographic Presentation

CALCIUM HYDROXIDE CEMENTS

MATERIALS	APPLICATIONS
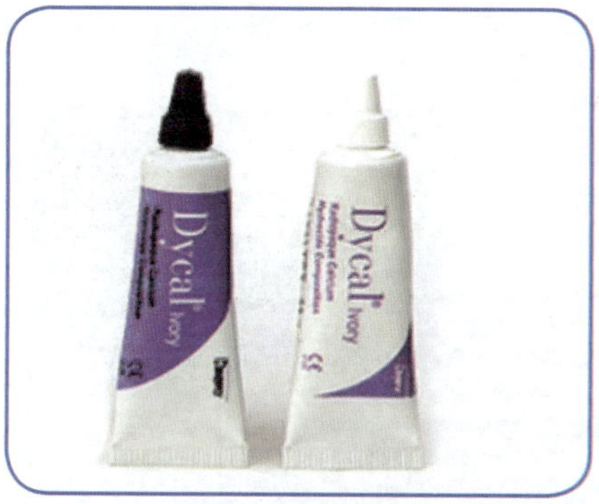 Fast Setting	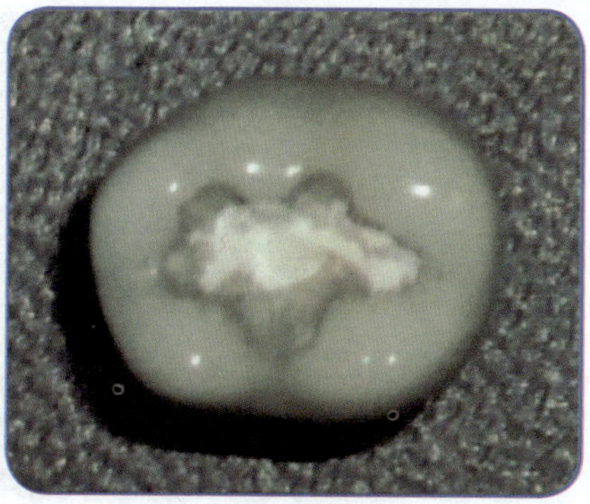 Cavity Liner
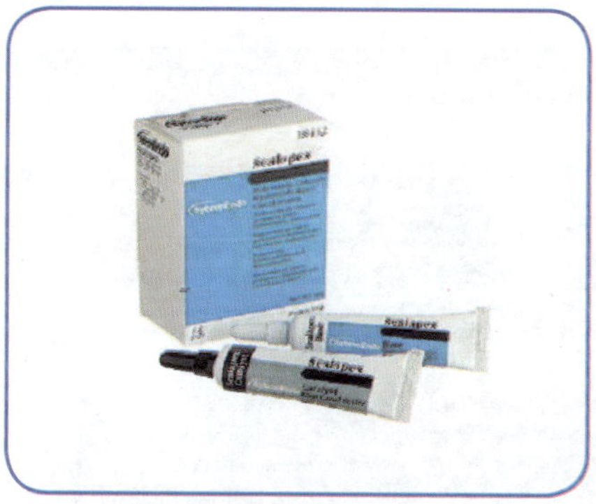 Slow Setting	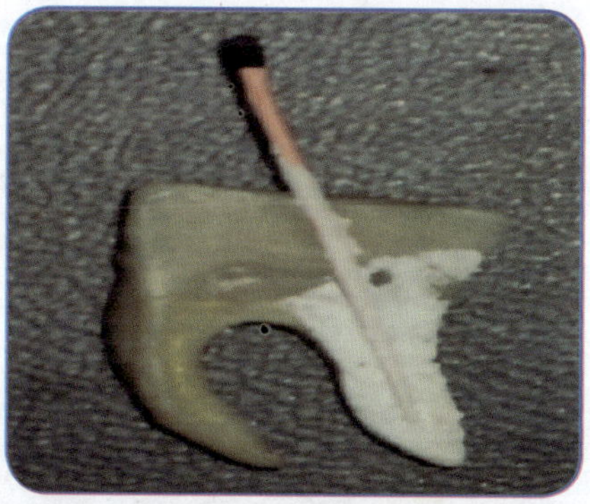 Root Canal Sealing
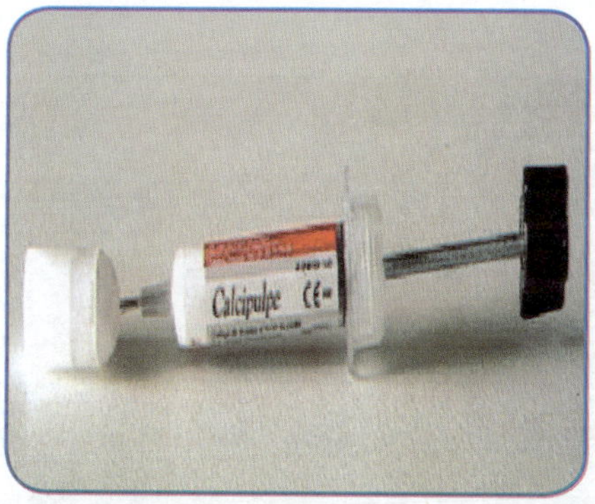 Non Setting	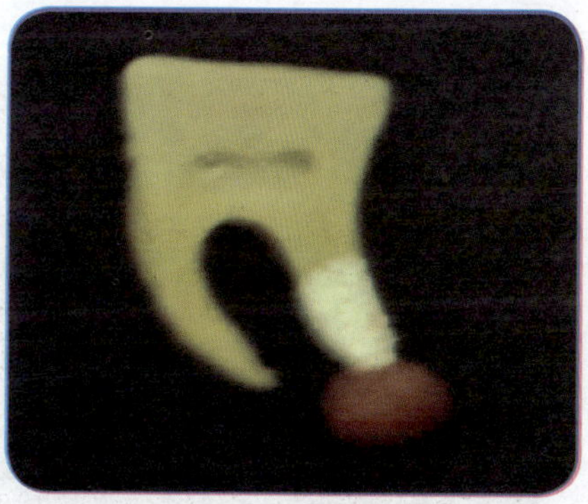 Root Canal Medicament

Photographic Presentation

INDIRECT RESTORATIONS

CROWN

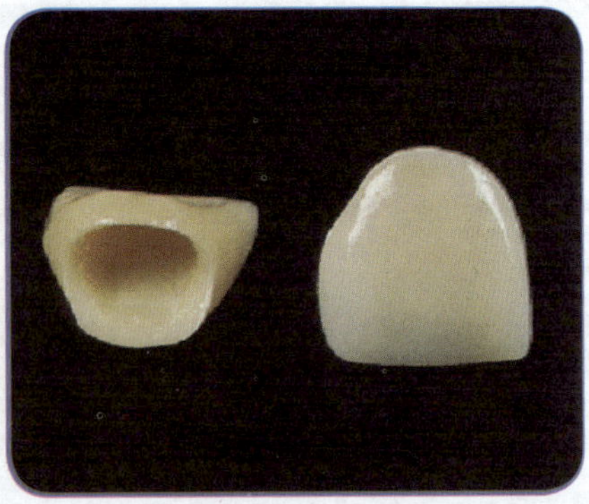

Porcelain Crown

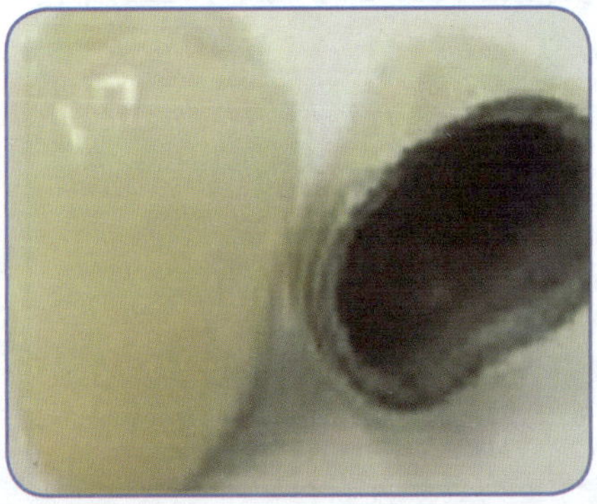

Porcelain Fused with Metal Crown

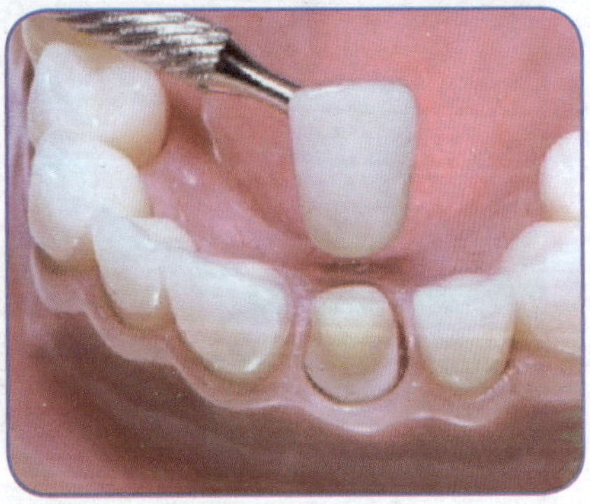

Placement of Crown

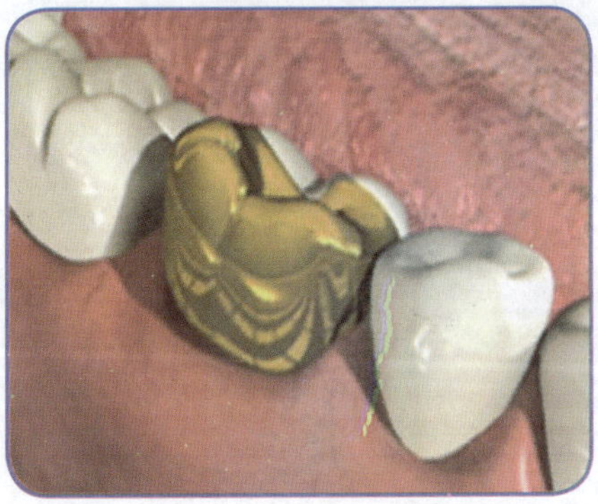

Three Quarter Crown

BRIDGE

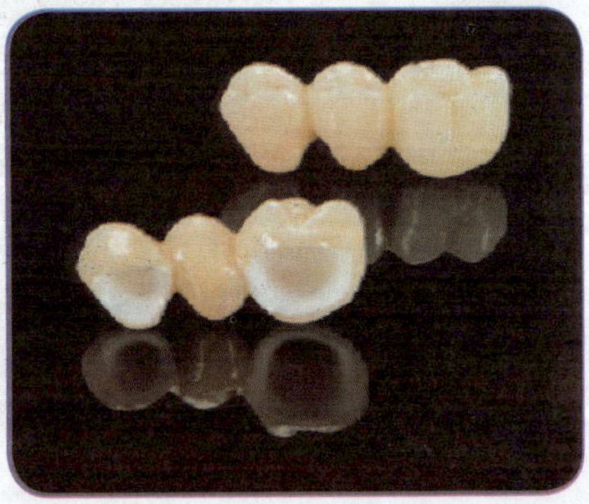

Porcelain Bridge

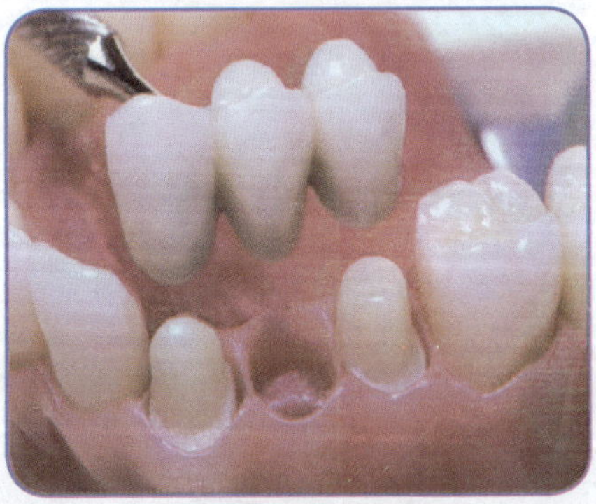

Placement of Bridge

Photographic Presentation

ONLAY

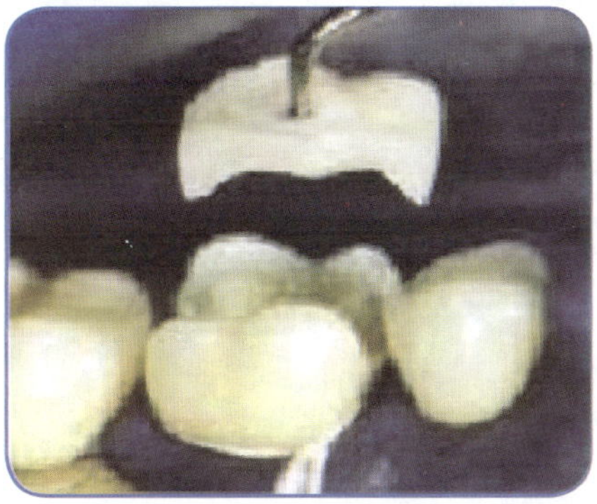

Before Placement

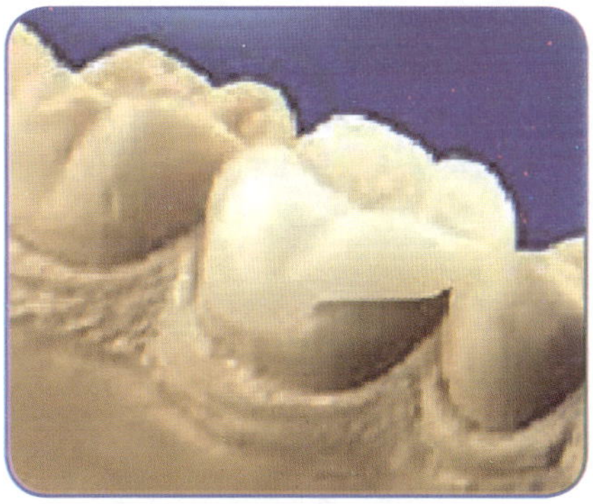

After Placement

INLAY

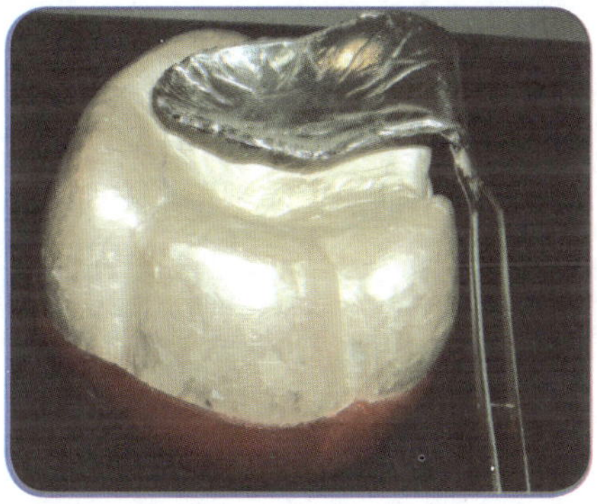

Before Placement

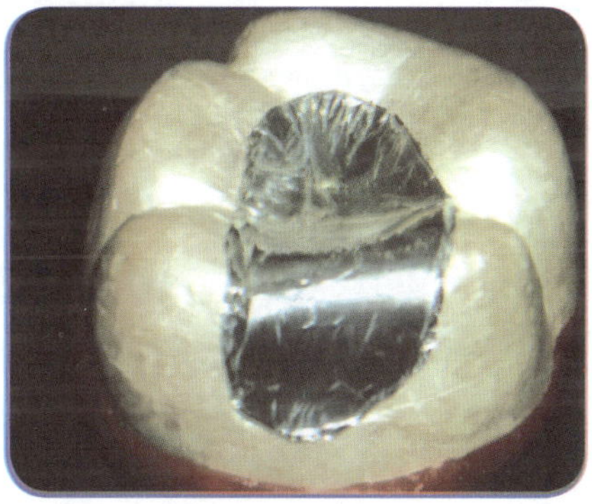

After Placement

VENEER

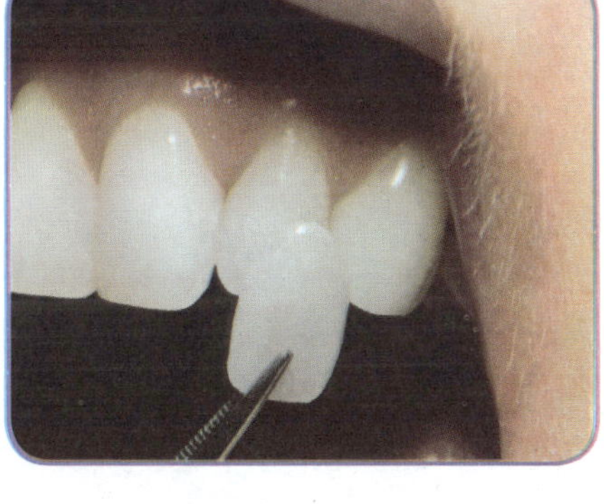

Porcelain Veneer

CERTIFICATE

CERTIFIED THAT

Mr/ Miss. ____

OF

______________ ***year B.D.S has carried***

out necessary practical work as prescribed by the

Department of ________________________________ ***for the year*** ______________

____________________ ____________________

H.O.D ***Instructor***